TOXIC
INTENT

TOXIC
INTENT

BRIAN HUMMEL, MD

Copyright © 2024 by Brian Hummel, MD.

Library of Congress Control Number: 2024925476
ISBN: Hardcover 979-8-3694-3397-3
Softcover 979-8-3694-3398-0
eBook 979-8-3694-3569-4

All rights reserved. No part of this book may be reproduced or transmitted in any form or by any means, electronic or mechanical, including photocopying, recording, or by any information storage and retrieval system, without permission in writing from the copyright owner.

Any people depicted in stock imagery provided by Getty Images are models, and such images are being used for illustrative purposes only. Certain stock imagery © Getty Images.

Print information available on the last page.

Rev. date: 12/09/2024

To order additional copies of this book, contact:
Xlibris
844-714-8691
www.Xlibris.com
Orders@Xlibris.com
861842

This book is dedicated first, and foremost, to Kristin. Your faith and support from our beginning has never faltered. You are my angel. To Christian, Stephen, Maggie, Sydney, and Jordan; you guys have all far exceeded a father's dream of being better than me. To Allison, Krissy, Asher, Kipling, Teddie, Amary, Hannah, Garrett, Sam, and Kathryn; you all make life fuller.

To Will, Norc, and Dan, the original storytellers. You guys inspire all who know you. Will, you are truly missed!

To my sibs, Brad, Becky and Barb, and Xavier and Jenni; you have been a part of it all.

To Tom and Sally Petcoff, Randy and Wendy White, Mark Pace and Darryl Pottorf, Mike and Nicole Cascone, Matt and Dawn Hummel, Andrea Davis, John Crites, Bekki Neal, and Roy and Nicki Carver—friends unwavering.

To the Gulf Harbour women's book club. Your encouragement is profoundly appreciated.

To the thousands of patients, I was privileged to care for over so many years and the staff that made us all look good.

Brian Hummel, MD
10/1/24

ADVANCE PRAISE FOR TOXIC INTENT

Dr. Brian Hummel's first novel, *Toxic Intent*, is a labyrinth of intrigue and fiction mixed with a megadose of cold, hard facts regarding China's trillion-dollar pharmaceutical industry and the lethal (also ingenious) potential of smuggling black-market fentanyl across the sleepy, wide-open spaces of Minnesota's boundary waters. The well-traveled Dr. Hummel, an internationally respected thoracic surgeon, knows the science. His characters convincingly share the specifics of what could happen—if it is not happening already.

Randy Wayne White
New York Times best-selling author

Toxic Intent is fiction, but for esteemed surgeon Dr. Brian Hummel, the story is a cautionary tale. It is a gripping thriller and a wild ride taking readers inside the world of black-market fentanyl and Asian cartels. Dr. Hummel has seen firsthand the tragic deaths of patients due to adulterated medications, born out of a desire for higher profitability and lax regulations. The story is disturbing, but in Dr Hummel's skilled hands, readers will also be entertained and educated.

Sanjay Gupta, MD
Professor of Neurosurgery, Emory University
Chief Medical Correspondent, CNN

AUTHOR'S NOTE

This book is one of fiction. Characters, events, and places are from the imagination of the author. Any resemblance to individuals living or dead is one of coincidence. While some locations mentioned are indeed real and can be seen or visited, the role in this fiction is that of benefit to the author and perhaps the reader. That fact established, I was provided the idea of the book from actual events.

In 2007–2008, hundreds of patients given heparin, a blood-thinning drug required to perform open-heart surgery and to treat or prevent a variety of medical problems, suffered a profound allergic reaction which included shock, and there were some resulting deaths. The author's awareness of this was firsthand, along with his partners in a cardiac surgical practice. Three patients undergoing open-heart surgery on a single day all displayed the consequences of shock as the heparin was administered. This prompted the notification to the FDA of our concern. We were visited within a day by investigators trying to discern the scope of the issues and its details. The cause, effect, and remedies to address the problem. The brief answer was that the manufacturer of the heparin was a China-based company. Not surprisingly, virtually the entire world's supply came from China. The biologic source was porcine, or pig, intestinal mucosa. The alternative source—bovine, or cow, lung tissue—had been abandoned because of fears of mad cow disease being introduced on a large scale to humans. The oversight of the Chinese producers was less than strict at the time. The attempt by the company to create more profit by expanding the volume of heparin with a cheap additive, chondroitin sulfate, was their solution to increasing profits. There were multiple deaths in the US arising from this, but the prompt reaction by the authorities responding to our initial call and the withdrawal of the suspect heparin saved lives. The effort to utilize bovine-based heparin is again being considered and encouraged, as the risk from well-controlled and -sourced herds of cows leaves little risk for the heparin-treated patient to be exposed to mad cow disease. A synthetic heparin is still commercially unavailable.

The incidence and consequences of physicians and other health care professionals suffering from stress and burnout has been well documented before, during, and after the COVID-19 pandemic. While the pandemic seemed to bring increased focus and attention to the problems, professionals have had a long and unfortunate history of substance use disorder. The symptoms associated with it include impaired control, social impairment, risky use, and the pharmacologic indicators of tolerance to and withdrawal from the addictive substance. The psychological impact on the professional of unaddressed stress easily leads to relief sought outside acceptable norms. The slippery slope of moving from having a cocktail on occasion to daily use and then to use of increased quantities to achieve the same level of relief is relived daily here in the US. The author's long surgical career brought to him on many occasions the opportunity to witness the devastating impact of unrelieved psychological stress and trauma, which manifests in such ways as suicide and drug and alcohol addiction. This book, I hope, brings further attention to this ongoing social and health care problem. It impacts not just the afflicted but also their patients, families, associates, and communities.

Finally, the epidemic of drug addiction, its origins, and its consequences to individuals, families, communities, and nations is well documented in many scholarly works. Frequent interaction with these suffering patients by me and my partners was necessitated by the infections of heart valves from intravenous drug injections.

Our practice reflected our county's growing crisis. In the fourth quarter of 2021, the county EMS responded to more than four hundred overdose calls. In that year, according to CDC data, Florida had over seven thousand eight hundred overdose deaths. The vast majority were attributed to synthetic opioids, the most common being fentanyl. This book does nothing to address this civic crisis, but it does perhaps highlight the problem for some to consider. While most fentanyl is coming through large ports of entry, the small amounts that can come across nontraditional sites are still a threat to all of our locales.

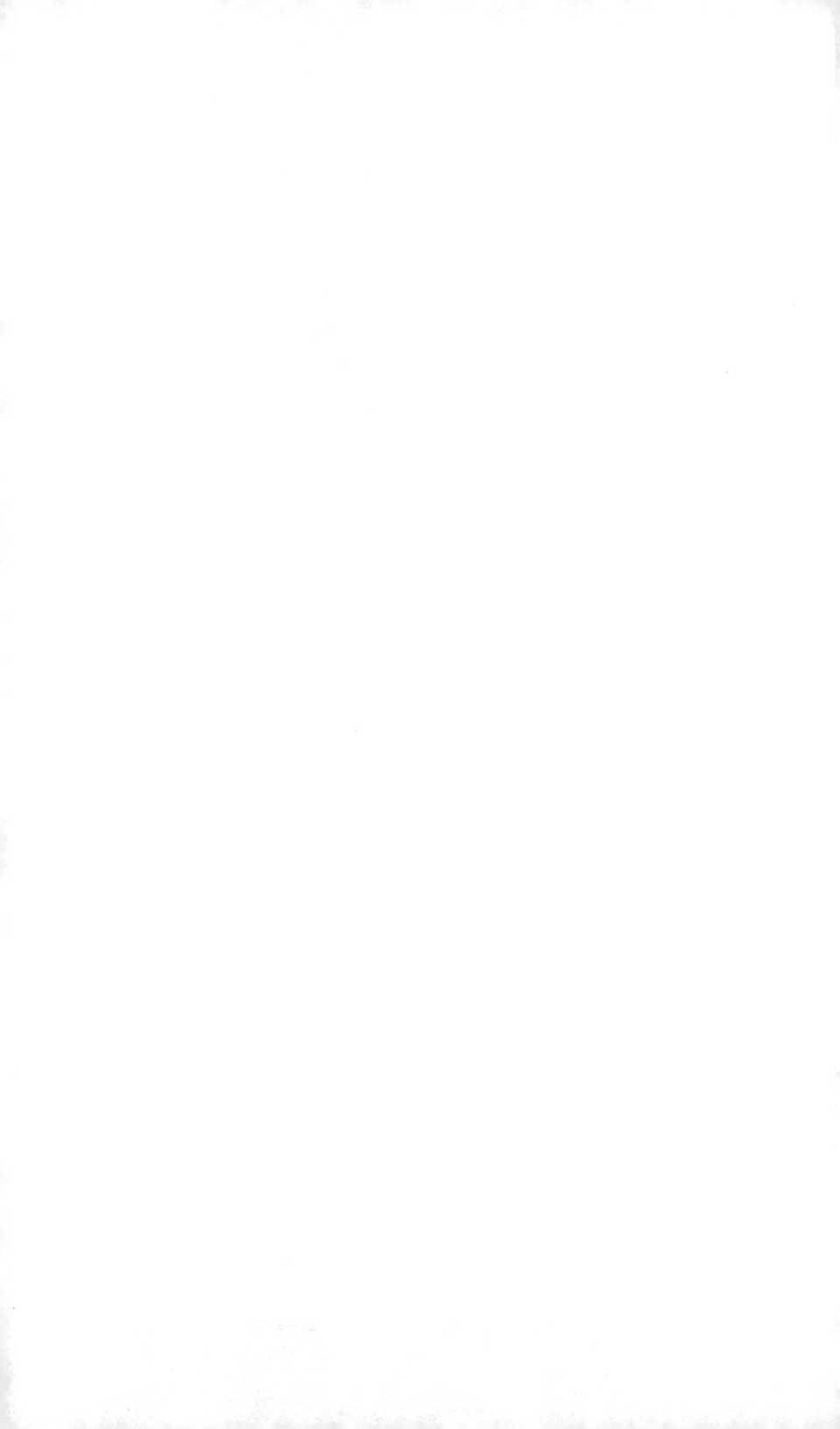

ONE

THE HEAT STILL felt oppressive. The high humidity had wrapped its wet sweater of moisture around anyone not within conditioned and cooled air. This single environmental solution allowed Floridians to remain attached to the reclaimed swamp they called the "free state," pandemic be damned. The condensation on my scotch glass dripped into my lap, creating an abstract map reminiscent of Florida—or, if considered in more sophomoric iterations, a flaccid penis drooping from the excessive heat. The last few drops off my glass fell into this virtual Gulf of Mexico near my actual physical location. The stillness and darkness were intermittently punctured by the low rumble of thunder and the flash of white summer lightning far to the west over the water. The horizon was distinguishable only when the vicissitudes of Zeus allowed us mortals to visually witness the charged atmosphere. Perhaps if I were adept at reading the signs, flaccid penis watermark juxtaposed to sharp strobes of discharging electrons, I would have noted that my tranquility was soon to be badly disrupted.

At that moment, it seemed my stress was evaporating with my ice—the cleansing power of a single malt over the multipronged pressure points of the day. It neared ten thirty, and I sat next to my backyard pool while trying to decompress. It had been a typical Friday of heart surgery: two valve cases and then a coronary bypass procedure that probably could have waited until Monday. However, the patient, the family, and the cardiologist were anxious—and understandably so, not just because of the patient's anatomy but also because of the waiting tension of the required procedure and the cost of a room at "Château the Hell with the Cost" hospital, where the meals were cold and resembled cardboard in any of the food group iterations offered. The beds were uncomfortable, the privacy equivalent to the suntan lotion dispensary on a nude beach, and the staff quality variable at best. Yes, it was twenty-first-century health care in the "civilized" world. Another two days of such anticipation would render Buddha to rethink his teachings of patience. With all these fine attributes, the price per night could still equal that of a new car. So, being understanding myself—and, if I dare say, the compassionate sort—I waited to get an open room in the OR for the surgery, sweet-talked and cajoled the staff to stay late, and proceeded.

This brought me to my current state of mental bliss for all the fifteen minutes I had been home. The best thing going at that point, besides the scotch on the rocks, was that I wasn't on call. There was real potential for getting a good night's sleep; reintroducing my out-of-shape, forty-five-year-old body to the gorgeous blonde who was my wife; and hitting the gym, in that order, over the next twenty-four hours. It seemed like a plan with no flaws. I liked both thoughts, as I had gotten out of shape by missing the last six days of my workouts—four-mile runs spaced every other day, with some weight training. This hiatus was the result of tendinitis in my knee. I did not want to exacerbate it with the running or the lifting. Perhaps this was the convenient excuse of a middle-aged jock. While I was out of shape in terms of my earlier years, I still tried to adhere to my routine, attempting to maintain my internal and external image of the athletic multisport athlete who left high school and walked onto a D2 football team as a defensive back. I certainly would not be confused with Ronnie Lott or Bob Sanders, but I was reliable, missed very few tackles, and always tried to make someone pay for traversing my assigned green space of the field. Wishful thinking and naivete dissipated as fast as my ice.

I had also maintained a fitness regimen as a consequence of being a prior marine reservist. I joined the reserves during the summer before med school. I wanted—rather needed—the monetary help, and I thought service was an important element of citizenship. I truly enjoyed it and chose the marines over the other branches as every marine is considered a rifleman and thus trained to be one no matter your MOS or assigned role in the service. I pushed myself to compete with the naval academy grad officers while at Quantico attending the Basic School, which all marine officers must do. It was reasonably grueling, but I took pride in besting the majority in the physical fitness tests. My training on the carbines, machine guns, pistols, and hand-to-hand combat gave me a rush. Learning land navigation, concealment, and platoon and company maneuvers was at times a lot of waiting, but it was fascinating to think in strategic terms. The live-fire exercises got your attention on the first go-around. I could have gone down a different path than that of a doctor intending to do heart surgery. I could have been—or at least my young self—enthralled with the military adventure. I realized the long time intervals between the adventures in the military would not have given me the daily rush that heart surgery provided. I continued going to the range to maintain my pistol skills and occasionally shot skeet as much for decompression as anything. I did not believe my home or family were in much jeopardy from gun-wielding intruders, and frankly, playing eighteen holes of golf took too much time. Shooting was quick, effective, and a great release of frustrations.

The phone rang, and while tempted to ignore it, I succumbed, as much out of habit as curiosity. Some habits should be broken. The voice on the other end was that of Tom Moore, my friend of many years. He answered to Tom, Tommy, or Tomboy, and I used them all. Tom was the partner on call for the weekend. I immediately girded for bad news regarding one of my patients, but the gravelly voice revealed that he was unable to be on call, as he was currently using his one allowed phone call from the county jail. "Ben, I need you to help me."

My initial response was "Nice joke," but his restatement of his location and the details that followed were about to alter my exquisite plans for the next forty-eight hours—and unfortunately many more than those first two days.

Tom and I had done our general surgical residency together at UT Southwestern in Dallas. During those five years together, we became good friends. He was the pied piper of our gang, and I was more the guardian of the little band of brothers that constituted our residency year group. He then went to Vanderbilt for his cardiac training, and I went to Iowa to get both vascular and cardiothoracic training. We remained close and talked frequently. Fortunately, we were able to find the opportunity in Florida to practice together. I had been best man at his first and second weddings. He managed to elope for number three, sparing me the obligatory duties. He stood up for me at my first, and thus far only, wedding.

As he described the situation, I found myself not surprised by his predicament. He stated he had been arrested because of erratic driving, a consequence of the girl in the passenger seat suddenly grabbing the wheel. Said passenger was not the wife of my Uber-driving partner. He claimed that to correct the course of his misdirected BMW, he was required to hit the girl to break her grip on the wheel. This blow was witnessed by the officer in blue who had been following the BMW since it pulled out of the parking lot of a local watering hole. Attendance at the watering hole while on call seemed like something that was normal for him, judging by his ongoing narrative. The blow did allow navigational control to return, according to Tom, but the bloody nose and small cut to the "hijacker's" cheek created a dark, wine-colored addition to the leather interior and her blouse. Ugliness all around. The visual impression of harm was not lost on the muscle-bound lad in blue once he approached the car. Thus, the erratic driving was compounded by a witnessed assault. Then, when questioned about alcohol consumption, Tommy, recalling some drunken sage saying, "Don't take the field test," deferred the opportunity to prove sobriety, thus in essence admitting to drunken driving. I'm not sure his interpretation of the law had been nuanced enough to understand that admission. He thus hit the trifecta of charges: reckless driving, assault, and driving under the influence. He was batting a thousand, and the game had only begun.

His misery was now to be shared with me.

I was trying to absorb the circumstances and implications of the events, and thus slightly disengaged from the drone his voice took on. His first request was understandable—that I come get him out of jail. But I learned that would not occur until the next day at the soonest. The next item was to get him a lawyer. This was followed by "Can you go get Emma"—Emma being Emma

Ridley, the victim of his Mike Tyson impersonation—"and make sure her nose is okay?"

His final desired gift on this particular wish list demonstrated a clear lack of reality in the mind of my now orange-suited friend and partner. "Don't tell the other partners about it."

I had always considered Tom to be a rational individual who could still be the life of the party. His red hair and freckles brought additional light to every room he entered. His ability to operate was probably the best of any surgeon in our group, drunk (not that I thought he had done so) or sober, and, to my estimation, one of the best I had ever seen. His Irish heritage, manifested by a gregarious personality, ever-present smile, and mischievous blue eyes, embraced all he met. There were no strangers in his life, only friends made—and those being made from the moment of introduction. Practicing with Tommy was one of the big attractions to my joining the group we belonged to. He operated like a magician, partied like a spring breaker, and subtly transitioned between the roles, never missing a case or a party. He was on his third marriage and was best of friends with wives one and two. Yes, everyone liked Tonny.

To complete my assigned and assumed duties, much to the chagrin of my scotch, my beautiful blonde former OR nurse wife I had to notify the hospital and answering service that I would now be on call for the weekend. I then reached out to a trial lawyer acquaintance and was educated as to the process and expectations of bail, follow-up court requirements, and the issue of impaired physician protocol to maintain a medical license. The road ahead looked less appealing to me, for both my friend and myself. If my jailhouse associate had been privy to what was being said, we may have had to put him on suicide watch, especially about the potential for meaningful felony assault charges in addition to the prospect of a prolonged program for "rehab" purposes. The lawyer kindly agreed to meet me early the next morning to reiterate our conversation. This was not how I saw the weekend going, even in a nightmare. As we discontinued our phone conversation, I noted that the electrical display over the gulf had seemingly been swallowed by the dark depths of the water. All that remained was the suffocating wetness of the night and a vague sense of dread I felt but did not yet recognize or acknowledge.

TWO

I CALLED TOM'S wife, Sue, and explained he had been pulled over and taken to jail on suspicion of driving under the influence. I avoided the details of the passenger and the assault. Sue, his wife of seven years, seemed only mildly disturbed. "I'm sure he will figure out how to beat this. I have some appointments tomorrow, so I guess I'll see him when I get home." She made no inquiry regarding obtaining his freedom. I was sensing a major fracture in the bond this marriage was based on. I suspected another ex-wife was in the making. I liked Sue but never understood the connection they shared. She was as antisocial as Tom was social. I would ask him when the time seemed appropriate, but assuming the duties of partner, not spouse, fell with a thud in my lap.

Dr. Self-Destruct, my partner of twelve years, had given me the cell number of his would-be hijacker. I contacted her to see how she was and to offer to evaluate her injuries. I knew Emma; all the surgeons did. Hell, the entire OR staff knew her. She was a perfusionist, the individual who runs the heart-lung machine, otherwise known as the pump, during open-heart surgery cases. She was an athletically fit woman in her thirties with long auburn hair falling to her shoulders, which was most often controlled in a bun or ponytail at work. Her being cute was only intensified by the way she filled her hospital-issued scrub pants and top. The top was nicely filled without spilling out, and the bottoms seemed to have been form-fitted as a green shrink-wrapped container filled with toned legs and an apparently very firm ass that emphasized the curves as she bent over the heart-lung machine to adjust the centrifugal pump heads. The scrubs fit as well as a custom couture Versace suit. This blend of genetic predisposition and obvious training commitment was appreciated by all in the room—straight, gay, male, and female. There were no detractors in attendance. She always seemed pleasant to me and was never caught off balance when an emergency or some extreme demands were made of her at the pump before and during cases.

She gave me the address, and I set off to retrieve her. The address took me to an upscale—nay—expensive condo complex steps from the Gulf of Mexico. I had a rough idea of the prices in the neighborhood and knew the salary of the perfusion staff. There seemed to be a disconnect between the two. Family money, ex-husband—who knew, but there had to be other income sources. I was mildly intrigued, but the focus of addressing and repairing the physical injury and mitigating an emotional and legal backlash was my immediate concern. She answered the door still wearing the blood-spotted ivory blouse and with an ice pack to her nose and eye. In retrospect I wondered whether the image of the bloodied blouse was meant to elicit compassion or make a statement as to the grievance of an injured party. Or was it simply not caring now how it looked or the message it sent?

I brought her back to my house, where the soothing words of my wife, Kay, would perhaps lessen any lingering ill will she might be feeling toward the guy who struck her. As we sat in the kitchen and I placed a few fine 5-0 sutures on her face and applied additional ice to a swollen nose (which fortunately maintained model-quality straightness) and eye, she described a different scenario than I thought I had heard courtesy of the jail's AT&T account.

"We were having fun, had a few beers and were headed to my place," she said. "I told him maybe we should reconsider, as he was married and all. Tommy then just lost it; he tried to punch me and caught me across the face. I started yelling at him, and he said to shut up or he would really hurt me. I was afraid and thought he would. But then the police pulled us over."

"Did you tell this to the cops?" I asked.

She hesitated before saying "I might have said he was very angry because I wouldn't have sex with him." It was at this point that I doubted the presence of my wife, or her soothing words, were going to be enough to alter what was beginning to sound like a shakedown or my partner's breakdown. I wasn't sure which slope we were headed down, but I did not want to step onto either of them. I also did not want to be the one bringing this shit storm accounting of events to Tonny or the other four partners.

The more we talked, the less convinced I was of the facts as presented by either of the participants. There seemed to be some unspoken subtext that neither party wished to share. I was at a loss as to what it was, and frankly was angry that it somehow was winding its tendrils around me.

THREE

I RETURNED EMMA, our newly designated maiden in distress, to her condo and drove home, lost in the bizarre tale of conflicting stories and now with questions that seemed to have no obvious, or in any event immediate, answer. I felt that while I was not in any way responsible, this unfolding tale of woe was going to complicate my life more than my unfinished scotch. The absent electrical display to the west was now being replayed on the horizons of my memory. The mental electrons delivering this personal storm were as powerful as the previously charged atmosphere, but only I was witness to this new brooding storm. This description of an angry Tonny seemed wholly out of character to the man I knew. Was it true? If so, what triggered it? His not getting laid seemed a feeble and frankly unbelievable incitement to anger, in my estimation. The night's stillness was interrupted by the croaking of tree frogs as I exited my car and lowered the garage door to the outside world.

The next morning found me rounding on the patients after very few hours of sleep, with the hint of dawn just cracking the ebony eastern sky. The irregular boundary of pale orange and blues tickling the horizon carried the first light and the promise of more heat and humidity. I hustled through the ICU patients and onto the floor to direct the arriving physician assistant as to the needs I had identified requiring attention. I simply stated I was covering for Tommy because of a family issue. It was vague but seemed to have enough truth to satisfy our employee. Leaving the hospital, I purchased some coffees and bagels and met the lawyer, William (Wyatt) Slife, with whom I had discussed the issues last night. We sat on a plain heavy metal bench outside of the marble edifice of the courthouse, the cornerstone of which was laid in 1915, according to the plaque next to our rendezvous site. Wyatt's physical presence was one of confidence, a regal bearing capped with thick gray hair, a pleasant face, and a silky voice that could lead any jury to find in favor for his clients. He patiently walked me through the hearing process that was to begin at 9:00 a.m. He predicted what the magistrate would say, based on the information I gave him and historical interactions with the state attorney's office. He felt they may not require a bond. I repeated the different versions of ride share fight night with Slife. He still felt, given Tommy's community ties and lack of prior involvement with the local constabulary, as well as his professional standing, minimal to no bail would be set. We had outlined the legal and practical moves going forward. This included the requirement of rehab for any licensed physician facing such charges. Wyatt emphasized to me, "You must get Tommy to understand the gravity of this. If he in any way tries to cut short the rehab as determined by the guidelines, his medical license will be but a fleeting memory to him!" He then added, "Tommy should not speak to his sparring partner. If he feels so compelled, a third party should be present."

A key part of the plan as envisioned by Slife was to quickly get Tommy entered into a postgraduate school for doctors and professionals (i.e., a renowned rehab center; he had two recommendations). He again noted that this was not going to be optional. He also stated that these "vacations" generally lasted three months or more. It was then he informed me he was going to leave me to attend the virtual hearing and that I was to call him if something other than this road outlined was put forth. He was on his way to the airport and would be returning in a few days. "This will be pretty straightforward; we should have Tommy back to work soon," he said while shaking my hand to leave. I somehow was brightened by his confidence. I didn't ask him about retainer money, nor did Tommy set a limit on the expense when he directed me to get a lawyer. I knew that no matter the cost, it was going to be covered by Tommy. As Wyatt walked away toward his apple-red Tesla, I once again felt that the burden of circumstances was pushing hard on my optimism meter. That brief respite I had just been feeling was lost to the morning sauna that was Florida in August. My next calls were to the partners to arrange a meeting for later that day or Sunday. I laid out the bare facts and the need to discuss how to manage the fallout and sort on- call responsibilities, given there were vacations and meeting times of others to be worked around.

Tommy convinced one of the jailors to loan him his cell phone. It turned out my partner behind bars had operated on a relative of the man, and thus a minor deviation from standard jailhouse rules was okay. My phone chimed a few bars from AC/DC's "Thunderstruck," the song frankly matching my emotions. I answered quickly, as is my usual response. (Pavlov's dogs have nothing on me.) "Ben, you must be sure I'm getting out of here. I don't think the partners will find out if I'm not stuck here. Is the lawyer here to make this happen?" Again with the distorted reality. No way the local rag of a paper would not be all over the booking and sundry charges being launched at my friend. I could almost see the bold print below the fold: "Heart Surgeon Beats Woman While Drunk." Hell, they didn't even need to involve Mothers Against Drunk Driving to incite anger and disgust toward this heart-mending but wayward soul. I also feared a less-than-comforting response by the hospital administrators—a group not particularly endowed with personal allegiance to wayward physicians. It was going to be a long day!

"Tommy," I replied, "Slife will not be there." The audible gasp and pause that followed spoke volumes. "He has explained the procedure to me and says you are to plead not guilty and that you have arranged legal representation. I believe he may have already spoken to the magistrate and requested your release with minimal or no bail. If they demand bail, I will secure the funds and pay it and pick you up. Slife also instructed me to tell you not to talk to anyone but him about what happened. Do you understand?"

His reply, while affirmative, seemed to have come from the hollowest of chambers within the human soul. I informed him there was a gallery Mr. Slife had told me about that would allow me to watch the video hearing. This seemed somehow to reassure us both. He would not feel alone, and I would see that the process was as predicted. I was accustomed to the orderly steps of my daily surgical activity. While this was not the routine of either of us, it was at least being presented in a stepwise progression. Unfortunately, some of the steps were going to be taken in the dark. I also informed him that Sue would see him later today, as she had previous appointments. He didn't seem at all surprised by his no-show spouse. I guess the pain of that slight was not accessible to his nerve endings.

The video proceedings began shortly after nine, and as the temperature rose outside, my anxiety behaved similarly as I sat in a small conference room, watching the newly accused and captured step up to a camera, hear the charges, and give pleas—all "not guilty."

Does anyone take responsibility for their actions? I thought. *Has the legal system deluded the entire populace into believing "not guilty" makes it so?* I cynically thought at that moment that the bar association had succeeded in the grandest marketing scam of all time. "Always plead not guilty; we can then milk the accused and the system of billions of dollars for legal representation." *What if more people simply said, "Yup, I'm guilty." No need for all the drama and wasted time. Let's simply get on with life,* I thought, but I realized I'm doomed as a pragmatist.

If the appearance of our citizenry parading across the fuzzy little video screen were meant to provide insight as to their transgressions, I believe all would have been convicted and sentenced without further ado. It is hard to overstate the impact of combining a hangover, no sleep, and the traffic cone impersonation the orange jump suit ensemble brings to the visual senses. I suspect that had I been in the same room, the olfactory impact would have served to magnify what was obvious—they were all guilty of something. In my head I could hear captain Steve McGarrett of *Hawaii 5-0* say, "Book 'em, Danno." Tommy's moment to shine did not occur until after ten. It was hard to believe a single night ridding the streets of our small town of the wayward souls I was observing left anyone else at large to foment more illegal activities. An officer observing the video pumpkin parade sat next to me. He had readily accepted the offer to share my bagels despite a belly that had already exceeded wide load parameters. Was I encouraging dietary indiscretion that would later find its way to my OR table? A question I avoided asking myself as he kindly informed me that the number of miscreants was typical for a summer weekend night. With all this real and potential monetary restitution to be paid, I wondered why our taxes were needed for any additional causes.

Tommy was finally visible in the orange (albeit monochromatic on the cheap monitor) conga line of men and women. When his turn to address the camera came, I sadly thought he looked no better than any of his mates of this current casting call. The voice of an unseen prosecutor read the charges: "Driving under the influence, reckless driving, damage to public property, assault and battery, failure to stop at a light, hit and run, and the coups de grâce, resisting arrest and assault on a police officer." At the conclusion of this litany of crimes, I must have looked as bad as Tommy. What the *ef* had just happened? Where was the simple DUI and maybe the inadvertent hand-to-head contact? The glaring "up charging" from what information Tommy and the girl had provided seemed Kafkaesque. I felt as though we were stepping though the looking glass, and it was very unsettling. Where was Slife? I must have missed the part when he explained how accusations from the state attorney's office were not the sticks and stones that break your bones, but damn, these words seemed to hurt me, and I wasn't wearing orange.

The magistrate didn't bat an eye, at least on camera, at what seemed to me to be some serious shit being flung toward my partner. To Tommy's credit, he maintained his composure, though I subsequently learned he hadn't really heard the charges, as he was simply focused on the face of the magistrate in the camera. The county attorney wanted significant bail to remind the accused of the seriousness with which their office took such matters. Bail was set at ten thousand dollars. This was going to delay Tommy's walk into the sunshine, as I had to get a bail bonder to post the bail, it being Saturday and thus there being no bank access. Not surprisingly, there were a number of offices containing bondsmen within several hundred feet of the courthouse. This convenience was not lost on me or the flock of like-minded friends and family members of those individuals seeking to loosen the restraining grip of justice on their physical bodies. I forked over a thousand dollars, which was nonrefundable, in the first office I walked into—that of "Bob the Bail Bondsman," as the signage read. I suspect the alliteration was lost on most of his freedom-seeking clients.

I will say that the décor of the office left one wondering what they did with all the nonrefundable cash. It was not used in making the office in any way pleasant, and I suspect some of the cash did not make the annual tax return filed from this less-than-Fortune-500 company. There was a wall calendar that could easily be referred to in confirming upcoming court appearances. Ashtrays last emptied during the Obama administration were adjacent to the gray plastic chairs in the all-in-one reception, waiting room, and office area in front of a chipped Formica counter. The heavy odor of burning tobacco enhanced the occasional plume of cigar smoke from somewhere in the back. I briefly wondered if it would be inappropriate to try and work a trade for future coronary bypass work for a bond today. I was certain Tommy would approve but recognized that the time to negotiate such a trade in services would require my extended presence in this environmental disaster.

Frankly I was willing to pay any amount just to get to fresh air. Perhaps they were smarter than I was giving them credit for.

I also half expected a wild-haired over muscled goon to be introduced to me so I would be compelled to help Tommy keep all his court appointments. While I didn't meet one, I feel certain the bounty hunter was available if needed. Perhaps it was the unseen originator of the cigar smoke. It would have fit.

FOUR

BY THE TIME I got back to the courthouse and completed the requisite paperwork, it was after 2:00 p.m. Tommy walked through the doors smiling as if he had just seen the Allies going down the Champs-Élysées in 1944. He felt liberated! I asked how his bed was, and the food, both of which received less-than-glowing reviews from this Michelin guide imposter. I offered to buy some lunch and stated we needed to talk about next steps. I also mentioned he should contact his wife to eliminate any worry about his absence. He said that was not needed, as she never questioned his whereabouts, and that frankly the marriage was nearly terminal at this point. My ultra-keen prescience was again confirmed. These facts I had accurately gleaned from the conversation with Sue the night before. I tried to act moderately surprised and expressed my honest sympathy. "No need to sweat it, my friend; it's for the best," he replied. The day's news just continued to evoke mixed reactions from me and, as near as I could tell, no real concern on the part of the accused.

We entered a beachside burger joint, where the smoky aroma of grilled cheeseburgers pleasantly collided with the heavy salty beach scents of water, sand, and coconut-infused suntan lotion across the narrow strip of a colorful beach-toweled garden blooming with bronzing bodies. We proceeded to find a quiet table in the corner of the small establishment more suited to the tourists than the locals. This was my intent given the frequent encounters with old patients that occurred when going about daily activities in our smallish town. This popular winter destination's population expands by 25 to 30 percent between Thanksgiving and Easter. The Midwestern snowbirds creating a migratory hell of clogged roads, with drivers turning across three lanes of traffic after suddenly determining the Publix grocery store would somehow vanish if they were required to proceed to make a U-turn under some semblance of control and within the dictums of rational and proscribed driving laws and etiquette. I felt our small town inexorably slipping into the realm of memories that I had always attributed to my grandparents: "Things just aren't the way they were when I was a kid." We were experiencing the problems always associated in my mind with the big cities. The traffic, increasing evidence of drug use and its criminal element, the recent discovery of a human trafficking ring on the outskirts of our hamlet—yes, all signs pointed to growth unfettered. Asphalt and concrete spreading like a malignant rash into the wetlands to our east and moving west as far as the gulf water's edge. The very thing that was attracting the people was being destroyed with every U-Haul and moving truck that disgorged its northern-impregnated contents on the doorstep of a vanishing paradise.

 The waitress eyed us as locals, given our absence of bright floral shirts and flip-flops. I suspect her quick assessment of potential tip size was correlated to the gaudiness of the shirts and shorts of the patrons. She efficiently took our order of a couple of burgers and fries. I noted that Donny avoided ordering a beer, and he said that given the night's debacle, he was not going to drink for a while. I congratulated him on this little declaration and concurred with the motive being valid. I was not quite ready to discuss the mandatory rehab stint as a requirement for maintaining his medical license. I felt the subtle mixture of greasy fries and bargain-basement hamburger would improve my delivery of perhaps nauseating news to my friend. I then revealed there was to be a partner meeting the next afternoon. He looked at me as if I had personally attempted to destroy his career. "Why did you tell them? This is all going to go away quietly," he insisted, his voice now rising above the strains of Jimmy Buffett's "One Particular Harbor" and the apropos lyrics: "But now times are tough, I got too much stuff. Can't explain the likes of me." Tommy captured by song! I saw anger and disappointment in equal measure as a cloud crossed his face and his eyes were seemingly lost in a future vision, I was not privy to. I explained that the group was absolutely going to find out and that being up front with them was not only the right thing to do but was the only reasonable action he could take if he wished to remain in the practice and the community. He remained silent for a moment and then said, "I get it, but I still wish you hadn't told them." It was at this point that our conversation was given the slap of reality. Tom's phone rang, and he answered. "This is Dr. Moore." His face lost enough color that the freckles seemed to fall off, and the palest of white remained. His blue eyes narrowed, creating creases at the corners. "I have no comment" was his next statement, and he clicked off the call. "The paper wanted my statement on the charges and wanted to know if I had assaulted others besides Emma and the officer in the past," he said, his voice now so low that the floor, sticky with a sheen of unknown burger condiments, caught the words clearer than I. The mayo-enhanced floor adhesive refused to release his voice back to table level. It was just as well, for the pain of the soon-to-be focused news and community spotlight was going to swallow more than his voice.

Surgeons are frequently and not unfairly dubbed "narcissistic." This label is even more frequently assigned to cardiac surgeons. Narcissists can live comfortably in their own self-created worlds. I knew both Tommy and I, as well as three of the other four partners could, on any given day, display classic traits of the disorder. But I felt Tommy was not creating his own facts or reality now. He was confused as to what he was being presented with. I paused and then said there was more information from Slife I needed to share with him prior to the meeting. First, there were the unexpected charges of resisting arrest and assault on a police officer. This seemed to catch him as if hearing it for the first time even though the charges were clearly stated at the video hearing and by the reporter minutes earlier. "I didn't touch any policeman or -woman. I did not resist; I simply tried to explain I was a surgeon on call, and could we just forget the whole thing?" While his words seemed earnest, it felt as if there was more to this than he was going to share. The waitress returned to refill our Diet Cokes and then tried to perhaps capture a larger tip with a smile directed at Tommy. I thought that interesting, as he really did look like he had not slept and had been in his clothes a day too long. Go figure. Sex appeal under cover. Tommy didn't respond to this subtle siren call—a clear indication of his mental state.

Having consumed the fries and most of the cheeseburger, I felt ready to continue. My next bit of educational information from the lawyer was regarding the prolonged and mandatory sabbatical he was to go on to maintain his license. I shared the minimum three-month number that was given to me. This, I explained, also dictated the need for the partners to be involved. The confident "I did nothing wrong attitude" evaporated. I could see this was not the "one particular harbor" either of us sought. It was closer to Jack Johnson's "Losing Hope." We sat for a bit longer as I tried to address his questions regarding the process of rehab, choosing a facility, and when to start. On the first two, I could only offer the couple of anecdotes I was aware of and that there were only two really good programs as far as I knew—the one outside of Atlanta and the other in Minnesota. I then offered that Slife had suggested that Tom identify the program and get there as soon as possible (i.e., leave on Sunday or Monday at the latest). All the court proceedings would be put on hold, and the court would look favorably on this proactive attempt to get his life under control. I could sense that the ship bearing his personality and soul was already taking him into waters neither of us recognized or had in any way charted. The sudden stillness and quiet between us was like watching the shore slowly slip beyond the horizon as his emotional sloop eased away from me, the room, and the life he had been living. I was aware it was happening and understood that the cargo of his life, if returned, would be forever altered in texture, no less than the scars we daily put down the center of our patients' chests. We parted with my dropping him at the impound lot of the county sheriff. He wanted to retrieve some things from his car and would Uber home, as his driver's license was automatically suspended pending the outcome of the DUI charge. I again confirmed the partner meeting at four the next day.

FIVE

I RETURNED TO the hospital and saw a couple of consults, one of which was going to require a valve replacement and coronary artery bypass on Monday. I could already see the impact being down one surgeon was going to have on the practice and, selfishly, on myself. More calls, more cases, more stress. I was struggling not to be angry at my friend. The other consult was for a young woman, twenty-two years old, suffering from endocarditis (infection of the heart) involving her tricuspid valve. While at this time she was not in need of surgery, she reminded me once again that the world of drug addiction and its consequences were now inescapable even in this formerly quiet blip on the edge of the gulf waters. This malady had been becoming much more common in our practice over the last two years. We had seen a large increase in the sheer number of patients with similar issues, and unfortunately many required open-heart surgery to repair or replace these infected valves. Some died from extensive infections and damaged hearts. An unsettling problem was the return of many of our "successfully" treated patients with recurrent infections due to a relapse. The safety net of adequate rehab facilities; doctors trained and willing to provide medically assisted treatment; and the sheer volume, cost, and time to care for those suffering exacerbated the problem—and not just in our tiny universe, but nationwide. Perhaps the excesses of money, greed, and good times was simply too strong an attraction to expect a reprieve anywhere humans congregated—this town proving no exception.

Sunday morning following rounds, I called to check on Tommy and got no response. I was not particularly surprised but wanted the reassurance that he was okay and making some plans regarding rehab and prepared to face his partners. I thought I would also check on Emma to see how her injuries were resolving and to get a sense of whether she was inclined to make the issues facing Tom any more complicated. I would have called but was near the condo complex I had retrieved her from and returned her to in the early hours of Saturday morning. The parking lot again spoke of money in the retinue of expensive autos gracing the shaded concrete resting place of the mostly foreign-labeled land chariots: BMWs on the low end, a sprinkling of Ferraris and Lamborghinis at the other end. I again was curious as to the background of our perfusionist.

The door to her condo was ajar and opened wider with my knock. "Emma, It's me, Ben. Are you home?" The silence was punctured by the distant soft roll of the gulf waters on the beach in front of the condo. I was debating further advancement when the sight of the bloodied blouse she'd worn caught my eye on the floor. Next to the ivory and blotched, red-stained Milano silk garment was a pool of fresher blood that spoke of more than my suture repair being disrupted. The ferrous scent of blood, well known to my olfactory tract, filled the condo. Again, the response of a surgeon to fix the problem propelled me through the door and down the short hallway to a great room holding a less-than-welcoming scene of a struggle. A lot of blood, broken glasses, pictures on the floor, overturned chairs, and no combatants. No one for me to administer aid to—and for that I was grateful and immediately disturbed. Who had fought to at least near death, and where did they go? I suspected the police would soon be asking that question of anyone who was within earshot. I stepped back out to the hallway and toward the door. Before exiting, I tried to investigate the kitchen and office space of the first floor. I touched nothing, recalling all my TV training from one of the multiple NCIS venues. While briefly debating the implications of calling the police, I looked around for security cameras and was surprised to see none that were obvious near the entry to the condo. Given the insurance premiums accumulating in the parking lot, I was certain cameras were capturing the comings and goings of the denizens of the enclave.

I made the call. I described the scene I had stumbled on and stated that, as a doctor, I was concerned that the amount of blood that appeared to be no longer circulating within the host's body would leave one to wonder about said host being available as a potential voter in the next sheriff's election. At least I think that's what I tried to say; the dispatching individual seemed more focused on who I was, how I came to my conclusions, whether I was invited in, and such. A short time later, a cruiser pulled in and disgorged a twentysomething wannabe badass Chuck Norris who unfortunately more closely resembled Barney Fife. I led the young officer to the threshold of the condo and explained how far I had entered and what I had seen and not seen (i.e., no bodies). He entered the hallway with his gun drawn and proceeded beyond my vantage point as he turned into the great room. I heard a muffled retch, and the paler version of Deputy Fife reappeared. I asked whether he had seen a body, given his audible and visual response, and all he got out was "There was so much blood." Again, I was feeling relieved, but I was also unsettled with the need to yet again wait for a more senior officer to respond and choreograph the next steps in addressing the question of whose blood this was and where the players were.

The morning stretched into the afternoon as I repeated my version of events to yet two more individuals from the local police and the county police. Apparently, the condo complex grounds straddled jurisdictional boundaries of the two agencies, and rather than cede investigative control, they would simply duplicate efforts and time, as well as taxpayer funds, until the higher-ups figured it out. This efficiency did nothing for my mood or my confidence that either one was capable of logical processing or taking an investigating direction that might lead to the victim or perpetrator. Somehow, only after hours of slow-motion interrogatories, they got to why I was there and what my relationship was with the condo resident. Their questions were easily answered, but I knew the association of checking on our work associate could lead to the injuries sustained in the assault report they had not yet connected to Tom. I perhaps oversimplified by stating she had had some minor surgical procedure and I thought I would check in. I quickly deduced that if it went further, I would play the doctor–patient confidentiality card, but it wasn't needed. I guess curiosity was not the strongest character element driving these officers. I had resisted the urge to again call Tom until I was released from the cone of inquiry and escaping beyond the crime scene tape separating the condo from the parking area now flush with overcooked sunbathers, passersby, and media trucks. I so wanted to be invisible, but my luck would simply not grant the power to me. I was about three steps from my car when a local reporter shouted, "Hey, Doc, what's going on?"

My first response was an accurate "I'm not sure; I guess you will need to talk to the authorities." I knew there were going to be follow-up questions, so the next response was less than accurate. "Sorry I can't chat; I need to get to the hospital." I quickly closed the car door and exited stage right. What the hell was going on?

Once a couple blocks away, I redialed Tom, courtesy of Bluetooth. As the dial sounds filled the interior of my car, the equally disturbing cerebral static filled my brain. Tommy answered his call before I answered my skull-encased dial tone. "Hey Ben, I saw I missed a call. Sorry, I was on the line with the Hazelden-Betty Ford center." The renowned treatment center for addiction I knew. "Working on my admission intake for rehab."

I felt a sense of reduced pressure that I was unaware had been expanding with in my chest for the last couple hours. "That's great," I replied, and quickly followed with "Have you been in contact with Emma?" He stated he had called her the previous evening and apologized for the whole incident and that he was going to be going to rehab to try and atone for his deficiencies and their impact. This again sounded like a minimalization of reality, but I wasn't feeling this was the venue to embark on that discussion. "Tom, what time was that?" I asked.

"Around midnight, I think. I had a long discussion with Sue about where our marriage was and what she wanted. In the end, we seem to agree the marriage is on fumes and that my spending time in rehab to reprioritize was probably a good thing."

I told him I thought that was the right direction as well, but again the failure to address the elephant in the room—evidence of alcoholism—seemed a glaring blind spot. I asked if she, Emma, seemed okay or whether anything was unusual other than the need for the call in the first place. To this he responded "No, but why the questions?" I told him of the scene in the condo and that I suspected the police would be contacting him shortly to see if he had any information about the affair. A long silence followed, and Tommy then offered, "I think she may have been involved in something illegal, but I have no idea what or with whom."

I figured this was a good time to invoke the "the less I know, the smarter I am" mindset and urged him to contact Wyatt Slife, his attorney, and tell him his suspicions and how to answer the questions that would be rumbling toward him shortly. "You are going to the partner meeting, aren't you? If you need a ride, I'll come get you." He assured me he would be there, and Sue was going to drop him off. "That's great, and I'm glad you are going to speak to all of us at once. From what you said about Hazelton, I presume you are ready to get started. Any idea when?" I was trying to temper my own growing anxiety about the supercharged atmosphere enveloping my little world.

"I leave tonight directly from our meeting. Sue is taking me to the airport, and somebody from Hazelden will meet me at the airport in Minneapolis"

"Sounds like a plan, my friend, and I'm proud of you for taking this step. I'll see you shortly at the meeting."

Interestingly, as we concluded the call, the serenity prayer came to me: "God grant me the serenity to accept the things I cannot change; courage to change the things I can; and the wisdom to know the difference." While I drove, I hoped these few words would stay with me, as I felt I was going to need them.

SIX

THE MEETING WENT as well as I could have hoped. In the end, we stated we were glad Tommy was getting help and that we as a group were concerned for his drinking. Unstated were the associated public rumors of drinking on call, now confirmed by events. We all pledged our support and mentioned that he needn't worry about his paycheck or job status. While his paycheck was one thing, there was no firing an employee, and that's what we all were, protected under the Americans with Disabilities Act. Alcoholism is on the protected list. I think we sounded more compassionate than some felt individually.

Throughout the meeting, I did not disclose the bloody scene at the condo, my questioning by the police, or my growing apprehension I felt about our future. I had no good reason to not offer this information, and I frankly should have to protect against the potential bombshell revelation I expected would be coming. There simply seemed to be some dark force propelling us to a denouement no one in the room could foresee and I intuitively wanted to avoid. We sorted out the ramifications of being down one surgeon, how the scheduled cases of Tom's would be addressed, and the all-important preservation of our vacation time. The mood in the room was complicated by self-interests, patient interests, and the desire for a friend and colleague to get help while suppressing an "I knew this would happen sooner or later" retrospective. The subtle narcissism that we could not suppress would have delighted the therapists we all should have had on speed dial.

The meeting broke up after Tommy departed for the airport. The requisite glass of wine was consumed, and the post meeting analysis was completed. We congratulated ourselves on the compassionate response we displayed and the forbearance in not name-calling our partner. All the while, my compartmented memory of the bloody condo was not brought into the sunshine of the group. I wondered as to my subtle paranoia keeping me from disclosing the facts. I really should find a therapist!

My drive home was interrupted by a couple calls back to the hospital to answer a few routine questions and to establish the now shuffled operative schedule for the next morning. Completing this, I received a call from "unknown caller." Again, I can't help but answer. The gravelly voice responding to my somewhat agitated greeting was succinct and threatening in tone and tenor without saying anything overtly threatening. "Just be a fucking doctor. You don't need to be anything else." While such advice is contrary to those of us trying to prove to ourselves that we are more than just surgeons, I didn't believe this little piece of self-help new age wisdom was intended to alter my spiritual inclinations. The phone clicked off, and I drove on toward the setting sun in the gulf. The subtle loss of daylight and clarity, afforded those in the light, was unconsciously ruminating within me. I was heading down a path for which I was unprepared. Somehow the darkening horizon was again portending my coming dawn.

SEVEN

I WAS OUT of bed before 5:00 a.m., unable to push aside the colliding thoughts and necessary actions I would need to complete today. My understanding spouse rubbed my hand as I tried to quietly exit the bed. I had told her of the bloody scene at the condo and that I had not shared the information with my partners. While she didn't understand my reluctance, she nonetheless said I would do the right thing. I'm not sure the endorsement was based on faith or optimism, but at least I felt as if I had told someone besides the police. I did not share the phone-delivered advice to "just be a f'ing doctor." This, I felt, was an unnecessary burden to her. This confessional time was quickly followed by a brisk lovemaking session that had been postponed from Friday night. With tired eyes, a common malady in my profession, I made my way to the modern kitchen that, in its shining glare of stainless steel, granite, and glass-fronted cabinets, felt alien to me this morning. Assuming the burden of the unpredictable and unwanted quickly altered the acuity of day-to-day observations. I started the coffee and trudged in old-man-like fashion to the driveway to retrieve the paper. While the story was not the lead, the prominence of the article describing a local cardiac surgeon arrested and facing multiple charges, including assault and battery, resisting arrest, and DUI, seemed to be screaming to me from the front page. I was grateful Tom had departed yesterday and, God willing, was cocooned in the confines and protocols of rehab, thus keeping the harsh and damning verbiage from his visual cortex. I thought that if I were in his shoes, this article would make me want to drink.

I read the article a couple of times and noted it did not mention his sparring partner. I guessed that was going to change once the description and location of the bloody condo story cleared the transom of the sinking local paper. Like all locals, the printed news was insufficiently producing revenue to keep them afloat. Unfortunately for Tommy the titanic moment had not yet scuttled the current edition of gotcha publishing. It seemed their most common editorials, exposés, overhyped headlines, and frequently misquoted or misinterpreted facts came from the local health care business. If you thought Monday-morning quarterbacking was bad, step into the administrators' and doctors' shoes for a while. An adverse event was "willful" neglect; a less-than-optimal quarter financially represented gross mismanagement, and a profitable one an example of runaway health costs due to greed. There was no middle ground, no objective evaluations, and no compromise. Their readers got the version and perspective of jaded, cynical reporters and editors who, even if young had encased their inquisitive nature in sensational impervious garments that, I suspected, were given them upon graduation from the Acme School of Journalism. Ruminating on this bias and my less-than-gracious opinion only darkened my tired mood. Damn, I hated Mondays.

I arrived early to the hospital. I noted, not for the first time, the near universal facade of hospitals constructed after 1980 containing modern stone or faux stone slabs across the front, separated by reflecting glass spacers that, when viewed upon entering, reminded the unfortunate patients and families doing so of their compromised status as normally functioning entities. The unique vessels contained emotions, dreams, and memories of years, months, days, and hours, all before the integrated anatomic engine sheathed in their epidermal armor broke down in some fashion, the breakdown derailing the planned life trajectory they had crafted—if not in reality, at least in fantasy. This modern version of architectural repetitiveness had the same impact today as the earlier versions of stone and mortar had had on the minds of those entering in the decades before. Perhaps more of the afflicted walked out of these institutions currently, but the buildings themselves still held powerful forces of disease and contained the consistent promise of cure in conflict with death. The universal emotion of hope and surrender that filled all who entered was just as prevalent in the third-world hospitals and trauma units I had visited and worked in as it was in the cities and suburbs of the modern world. All of humanity, it seemed, did not want to conform to Dante's directive to "abandon all hope ye who enter here." No, we all want to hope. It may be that last thing we can embrace.

 I completed rounds, including Tom's patients and headed for the OR. The head perfusionist, Kirk, approached me at the scrub sink as I was preparing for a double-valve, coronary bypass case that had originally been scheduled for Tom. "Ben, have you heard? Emma isn't here today." Before I could respond, an operating room coordinator walked up and said to Kirk there was a policeman at the desk asking to speak to him before the cases started. Kirk's color changed instantaneously from the over tanned, weathered complexion of an outdoorsman to a full-sized porcelain mask any kabuki dancer would have proudly displayed. The change left me stunned and curious as to the exaggerated response to the request for a visit with the officer. I get uncertainty and "What have I done; how fast was I going?" thinking, but this was as if he had been sentenced to life in prison.

"Kirk, are you okay?" I asked.

He mumbled, "Yeah, fine. You may have to wait on your next case with Emma not here." He then forced his body in the direction of the office of the operating room manager.

My thoughts were quickly refocused with the yell from the operating room that they needed me in there stat, as the patient's blood pressure was tanking and unresponsive to the usual endeavors of tilting the head down (Trendelenburg position) and administering boluses of epinephrine. The patient had been intubated and prepped as the physician assistant had begun harvesting the greater saphenous vein, utilizing a videoscope to allow its removal with small incisions. This vein would then be used in the coronary bypass portion of the procedure. "What happened?" I said as I gowned and gloved.

"Nothing obvious," Ralph, the anesthesiologist, responded. He had returned to the room when summoned by the nurse anesthetists at the first sign of profound hypotension. "The rhythm hasn't changed, CO_2 return is normal, and we just drew some arterial blood gases to confirm oxygenation. We gave a small dose of heparin for the vein harvest, and shortly after that we were on the rapid down escalator of blood pressure."

"Give a gram of Solu-Medrol now and full heparin dose but use another vial!" I said as I quickly used the scalpel blade to cut from the top of the sternum to the bottom from skin to bone in one motion. We would deal with the skin and subcutaneous bleeders later. The need now was to provide full circulatory support by getting the patient on the heart-lung machine as fast as possible. Normally time would be spent stopping those bleeding vessels as one proceeded. Now getting to the bone, I was handed the sternal saw, and the bony plate no longer stood between me and the structures I needed to access. The pericardial sac around the heart was quickly opened, and the ascending aorta was directly in view, looking like a barely pressurized hose. I stabbed it high toward the neck, covered the hole with a finger, and then inserted the cannula that would return the blood to the patient after being oxygenated by the pump. I had the nurse across from me hold the cannula in place and quickly stabbed a hole into the right atrium. Again, covering the defect with my finger, I placed a large cannula with holes near its tip, which settled into the inferior vena cava, and additional holes that would lie within the right atrial chamber itself. "On pump," I directed, and "Give additional heparin in the pump to cover us."

The blood pressure remained resistant to the blood pressure–raising drugs of epinephrine, Levophed, and methylene blue. But slowly the BP came up. The question was whether to proceed with the surgery or stand here and wait for the hemodynamics to normalize. "How is the ACT?" I asked. The response from the perfusionist was that it was adequate to remain on the pump. I was grateful for this, as we could avoid switching to the alternative of argatroban to replace the heparin as a blood thinner. The requirement of a blood thinner was an absolute necessity of utilizing the heart-lung machine. The ACT giving us a time for blood to clot. Without the blood thinning effect, the patient's blood would clot in the tubing and filters, with death quickly following. The alternative to heparin, argatroban, was likely to involve additional hours of simply waiting for the drug to wear off and potential for excess bleeding. There was no reversal drug to give, unlike that available for heparin. The need to decide was mine alone. I pondered the dilemma and weighed the pros and cons.

I noted once again the loneliness and power granted to me, the surgeon, in equal measure. The rhythmic beeping of the cardiac monitor, the soft whir of the centrifugal pump heads as they efficiently withdrew the blood from this trusting somnolent man and returned it to maintain his life, fully oxygenated and chemically balanced for pH and elemental content of potassium, sodium, magnesium, and more. I could seek the advice of the anesthesiologists, the advanced providers, and even a partner, but the decision was mine. The consequences would also fall to me. If a success, the team would appropriately be acknowledged. If a failure, the team effort would be forgiven but the family and lawyers would be looking to me to justify the decision and consequences. This was my environment, the arena I entered almost every day, and I never felt I truly comprehended or could measure up to the trust given or the knowledge and skill expected. There was no magical or spiritual intervention within me. I recalled from my youth the verse in the book of James: "God doesn't make the decisions for us, though. He gives us the gift of free will ..." I needed the wisdom of Solomon and skills equivalent to those of Michael Jordan. "Okay," I announced, "we are going to fix this guy." The room seemed to get quieter as all focused on their tasks.

EIGHT

FAR TO THE north in a rustic cabin in northern Minnesota, the quiet was profoundly different. Emma was awakening. As bad as my day was, and the patient's, hers was trying desperately to equal or exceed our misery. Her head swirled in the fog of an evaporating drug haze. The room seemed initially cloudy, as if she had stepped into the mist of a high mountaintop. No discernable landmarks seemed to be visible, and the light suffused as if traversing heavy gauze drapes. The distorted objects before her were slow to take the shapes intended for their function. The small table and a chair slowly transformed from the initial boulder she had thought was before her. The potbellied stove emerged from the tree stump she was sure had positioned itself to her right. She came to understand her primitive abode was not her condo, and the air was distinctly cooler and much less humid as it caressed her bruised cheek and blood-crusted arm and shirt. Her legs were scraped, as was her shoulder. She recalled her condo door being pushed open as she approached it following a knock. Were there two or three people rushing in? The hand to her face and the blow to her head. The metallic taste of blood in her mouth mixed with a chemical. The sensation of blood on her side and the knife she had tried to push aside as it came toward her swiftly. The groan of the man trying to put something to her face. Had he been stabbed from her parrying motion to avert the knife? She took stock of her torso and limbs. All seemed grossly intact, but the pain of movement, including deep breathing, was evidence of a mugging she had participated in as the receiver, not the giver. She slowly recalled the previous blow to her face from Tommy as she tenderly fingered the sutures in her cheek. Hell, what was with her putting her face to everyone's fist!

She slowly stood, and the brief vertigo—drug related, she hoped, and not concussion induced—caused her to again sit before falling. Then she took her first unsteady steps, learning to walk like a twelve-month-old. Not that she remembered those valiant exploratory moments, but exploration is what she now proceeded to do. The limited excursion, as vital as Lewis and Clark's trip westward, required her to step only five times forward until she ran into the equivalent of the Rocky Mountains. Progress was halted by the log wall holding a locked door in the center of its approximate fourteen-foot span. The door was a dense wooden panel with rustic but heavy iron bands crossing at its midpoint and hinges equally heavy in appearance, these being countersunk into the wood. No screws were visible. The side walls of the room were also of logs, with one transom window high near the peak of the pitched ceiling, which was smooth tongue-in-groove material. It sloped from the front wall to the back, the height at the back being about nine feet, and at the front twelve to thirteen feet. She could see clouds and some tops of pine trees though the window, which appeared to be a Plexiglas-like material rather than glass. Whatever it was, the housekeeper must have been on vacation or didn't own a ladder to improve the view. She chuckled a little as she thought of a housekeeper in this primitive rendition of a cabin. It was at this point she realized there was a sink but no toilet in the room. A five-gallon bucket was in the corner. Her brief chuckle from the housekeeper vision now swiftly shifted to a pitiful moan of pain, depression, and fear. What had she done to get to this geographic location and emotional abyss in which she found herself?

The slow 360-degree turn she made revealed the remainder of her immediate environment: the bed with perhaps a three-inch mattress and scratchy wool blanket upon which she had been lying, a short wooden table upon which a ten-inch handleless saucepan sat, a plastic glass, a spoon, and an old-fashioned hand pump that probably predated the cabin, as it appeared to have been constructed around it. The window was open slightly, with the top separated from the frame a few inches and the bottom hinged into the frame. A soft breeze circulated the room and felt amazingly good—a small plus to her ledger.

Glimpsing some pine trees though the window simultaneously brought the scent reminiscent of Christmas, which suddenly deepened the depression she was in. She considered that maybe the "holiday blues," or seasonal affective disorder, weren't limited to the holidays. Her location was a mystery. She had once vacationed with a boyfriend in northwestern Montana, and the air felt similar with its coolness and heavy conifer-fragranced sweetness. Her recollection of the "Big Sky" moniker attached to the state and proudly displayed on the license plates of locals seemed to fail at the limited sky view she now held. The other reminiscent olfactory memory was of a family trip to Maine as a child. The beauty she imagined from those snippets of heavily pined forests only deepened the shading veil of sadness she was experiencing in this chinked log cabin. Wherever she was, she was certain it was not on the first lists of longitudes and latitudes where her friends, family, or authorities might be looking.

She was beginning to sense that her recent small business enterprise may have come with some severe unintended consequences. Somebody was pissed. Her current circumstances would seem to indicate an anger perhaps somewhat deeper than the pissed-off variety one would encounter, say, over a contested parking spot or a dog dumping in one's front yard. No, this seemed to be the pissed-off emotion one associated with spies, kidnappers for ransom, or sex trafficking. She briefly paused on the mental image of being a sex trafficking victim; it was simply too foreign to consider, and she quickly reconfirmed her underwear were in fact on and seemed undisturbed. But now that sex was floating in the chaos of her mind, it seemed to create a space to occupy, and it was not going to relinquish its seat. But what would come? Until she came up with a better alternative, this ugly thought was going to mock her sanity. She was repulsed by the idea of being raped and felt an anger of her own building and churning within her. The knife-wielding attacker she was remembering now indicated she was looking at the far end of someone else's anger scale. She had never witnessed or ventured onto the level of rage she had felt from the intruder and that was rising in her chest. Some yet-to-be-labeled villain and motive must be in play. Theirs was a serious game, and she didn't know her role or the rules but understood she would be participating.

Exactly who, why, and why her were not remotely clear. She returned to the little side hustle she and Kirk Larson were running. Yes, they were making a little money, but this reaction, if related, seemed far above what a few thousand bucks warranted. Kirk's idea was to buy and sell some of the drugs utilized with the heart-lung machine. He being motivated by an improved cash flow and the opportunity to locally address the "supply chain" shortage that seemed to constantly interrupt or limit the delivery of necessary drugs for providers of health care. The deal seemed straightforward.

Kirk, the chief perfusionist, had been on a mission trip to China to perform cardiac surgery in some of the outlying provincial hospitals. He noted that the drugs they were using were as effective as our US commercial products, with no apparent problems with the drugs or their supplies. The labels were nearly identical and packaged like our products. The most commonly required drug was the heparin, but mannitol and Solu-Medrol (these also being used to prime the heart-lung machine's fluid reservoir) were also packaged in nearly identical fashion to the American brands. Kirk informed Emma they could buy these products from his contact and the contact would ensure they arrived at the hospital receiving dock. The contract Kirk had for the perfusion services included the price of the US brands for these drug supplies—a significantly higher price, all understood. The operating room budget, being a separate line item from Pharmacy in the hospital's accounting ledger, thus paid for the "standard price" for heparin and other drugs received when Kirk supplied a "case list" and the amount of the drugs consumed. The hospital system cut the check monthly to the perfusion group based on this stated volume. The tracking and management of these few drugs were historically the responsibility of the perfusion team, headed by Kirk "Quick Buck" Larson. The small print of the contract stated that all vendors for products must be preapproved by the purchasing department or quality committee of the hospital. This caveat had not been checked on in many years, and since the product packaging looked nearly identical to the US brand, nobody in Receiving noticed, nor would they have without a careful side-by-side comparison.

NINE

I WAS JUST finishing the closure of the left atriotomy that had allowed me to repair the leaking mitral valve of the patient. This repair was done with a single Gore-Tex suture to reposition a prolapsed posterior leaflet of the valve and an annuloplasty ring to stabilize the valve apparatus from future enlargement and to ensure the leaflets of the valve were supported at their base. I was feeling good about the decision to proceed with the surgery and felt we had given the man the best opportunity to survive and thrive. The doors to the hallway opened loudly; I heard it over the current song on my playlist, "Signed, Sealed, Delivered," by Stevie Wonder. I loved the intent of those lyrics. The door noise was again bringing that *drip-drip* water torture I had been experiencing over the last forty-eight hours.

"Ben, the carotid patient of Dr. Fry just crashed. He thinks the patient needs to get on the pump for support." The message was delivered emphatically but calmly by the head nurse of the OR. Being the section chief for cardiac surgery brought me to the sharp edge of the knife, so to speak, when others felt the options available to them were inadequate; and on more than one occasion it was the deficiency of the attending, not the disease, that prompted the call. Dr. Tim Fry was not in the deficient category. The guy was good both mentally and technically. If he felt pump support was required, something was truly amiss. My other partners were at other facilities we covered, and one was in the office, seeing patients. The first day of improv due to an absent partner.

The patient I was working on had all the major work, closures, and connections completed and would need only to be warmed and the air removed from inside the cardiac chambers prior to weaning him from the bypass circuit. The patient was in Trendelenburg with the major deairing completed, and I removed the aortic cross clamp to allow the heart to receive warmed blood in the normal fashion through his coronary arteries and the single vein graft I had placed. I told the physician assistant to watch the patient while I quickly went down the hall to Dr. Fry's room.

Upon entering the room, I saw that the silent but choreographed dance of CPR was in process. There was the command of epi and calcium to be given by the anesthesiologist. It was delivered in the firm, authoritative tone that spoke of this not being his first foray into potential medical mayhem. There was no yelling, no panicking, just the efficient motions of the chest compression, the ventilator bellows with their soft hissing, and the scrub nurse opening a tray of instruments I might require in placing this unfortunate soul on the pump. "Tom, what's going on, my friend?" I gently inquired.

He had just completed a period of performing CPR and stepped back from the side of the table. "Not sure. I had the carotid exposed for endarterectomy anesthesia, gave the heparin, and within in a minute we were seeing blood pressures that looked like the Dow Jones of October '29. The pressure isn't responding to any of the pressors, and while better with the chest compressions, still not great."

I looked at Kirk, the chief perfusionist, who had responded to the possible crash on pump message. "Okay," I said, "let's fully heparinize with a different lot of this stuff. Kirk was already assembling the pump tubing as I spoke. Give some Benadryl and steroids if you haven't already." I then took off the gown I had been wearing and regloved without scrubbing. There was no time to step to the sink, so a quick handful of antiseptic foam was it.

I informed the scrub nurse we would quickly expose the femoral artery and vein so they could continue CPR uninterrupted. A single cut through the groin and a brief dissection with the scissors brought the artery into view. I introduced a needle into the artery and placed a guide wire through it, removed the needle off the wire and slid the femoral cannula over the wire and into the vessel, made the connection to the pump tubing, and ordered some volume of fluid from the pump to be pumped into the patient. This same dance sequence was then performed on the vein, albeit with a longer wire that was advanced to the right atrium of the heart. This was confirmed by the anesthesia team that was evaluating the patient's heart with an echo probe they had placed in his esophagus from his mouth as CPR was ongoing. Their expertise was greatly appreciated by me, as it allowed me to visualize the wire within the cardiac chamber. As I was doing this, I told the circulating nurse to get my partner out of the office and over here to manage one of these two patients I now had on pump. Simultaneously advancing the long drainage catheter over the wire, I removed the wire and made the circuit connection. "On pump," I commanded while making a circular motion with my hand. The pump heads rotated. Blood readily flowed out of the long venous catheter and returned through the arterial catheter I was now securing. This had all occurred in a brief few minutes.

"Tim," I said, "I'll let you decide about proceeding with the carotid, but my recommendation would be to come back another day. If there is a stroke from this low-pressure shit, you don't want it attributed to your operation." Kirk, the perfusionist, looked at me quizzically. "The other patient came to the operating room with a compromised heart, and the shock and recovery would be very difficult without a well-functioning one. This patient's heart was presumably good, so best to minimize all the additional factors they must deal with." The understanding immediately showed on his masked face. "Kirk," I added, "I want you to collect the emptied heparin vials so we can look at lot numbers. To have two reactions this profound in one day makes me think we got some bad juju or bad heparin. Like maybe an expired batch from low-bid pharmaceuticals." Little did I know how close to home I was hitting.

Tim had agreed to abort the carotid surgery and had started closing the previous neck incision he had so artfully created. "Tom, while you are closing and this guy is getting stabilized I'm going next door to get my patient off pump. If you have any issues, yell. I think Bob should be here shortly from the office to help get this one weaned off pump when things have come back to baseline."

Tim nodded and, as I was heading for the door, stated, "I owe you one, buddy."

"You don't," I replied. I then mumbled, "But thanks for the thought," as the door closed behind me. There was definitely something going on here that didn't make sense. The *drip-drip* of bad events was getting to be steadier.

I returned to my original room and appreciated that the vitals appeared steady. EKG looked good, BP was 110/65 on minimal drug support, and the open chest was not filling up from some bleeding source. The body temp had come up to thirty-seven degrees centigrade from the low of thirty-two we had cooled to. This intentional cooling was to minimize the demands the body had for oxygen. "How are you doing up there?" I asked over the drapes.

"Everything looks amazingly good right now" was the reply from the nurse anesthetist, sounding surprised.

I wasn't sure whether I should be offended or not at the tone. I guess, given the emergent "crash" onto the pump, her skepticism was justified. My narcissistic side wanted to say, "Of course it's all good," but I suppressed the urge. "All right then, let's free the man from this ugly anchor of a pump. He wants to live and dance again," I quipped, not knowing if the guy ever danced. "Let's turn up the tunes." The Bee Gees' "Stayin' Alive," with the voice of Barry Gibb, crackled across the airwaves of our workplace. "Bring down the flow on the pump. Let's take it to the barn," I commanded to the circulating nurse and the perfusionist. They had all heard it before and knew we were headed down the final straightaway. Much of the tension we shared in the room was lessening as we reached this benchmark of progress toward a successful case. I would be soon asking to hear "Back in Black" by AC/DC. These were the songs that, when played loudly, made even the damaged old hearts I customarily worked upon feel like beating strong and sticking around to resume their lifelong cadence after a respite on the heart-lung machine. The deep bass metronome being laid down by Cliff Williams would set the tone for this patient's future. These daily reminders that the human body could indeed take a licking and keep on ticking were a testament to something far beyond my skill set or scientific understanding. There is something powerful pushing us forward, be it to a good place or bad. The answer as to the question of which place we go to is to be revealed only when we are on the precipice.

TEN

I LATER STEPPED into the hall after discussing the outcome and expectations of the recovery course with my patient's family. "We replaced the aortic valve, repaired his mitral valve, and did a single bypass," I explained. "He is stable currently, but early in the procedure he dropped his blood pressure to critically low levels. We promptly placed him on the heart-lung machine, and this appeared to stabilize him. At this time, I can't speak about potential complications, including a stroke. That said, I'm hopeful he is going to do all right. His heart function looked good with the echo once we were off the machine, he is on minimal drugs for blood pressure, and there appears to be no excessive bleeding. We will have a much clearer picture when he is awake, which will not be for hours." I answered a couple of questions about the valve repair and the low blood pressure issue for which I had no real answers at this time and acknowledged their thanks and headed to Fry's room to check in. Bob, my partner, had arrived, and after about forty-five minutes on the pump, the patient's vitals stabilized. He had come off pump, and Bob was repairing the femoral artery and vein where I had placed the cannulas. "Bob, thanks for giving me a hand. Everything okay?" I inquired.

"Yeah, we're good here. They told me about the hypotension. You think its heparin related?" he asked.

"I'm not sure, but I want Kirk to get all the vials we used today so we can check the lot numbers," I responded.

"He must be rounding them up. He left the room fifteen or twenty minutes ago," Bob noted.

I headed for the operating room director's office. The walk down the hallway gave me a moment to contemplate this sudden convergence of events that had descended like a free-falling elevator on my rather busy but predictable life: Tomboy arrested and charged with multiple albeit related "crimes," the other party involved in my partner's self inflicted nightmare now AWOL, and then today's experience of sudden patient deterioration presumably related to administration of heparin. It was not obvious to me that there was a connection other than my life and good humor being sorely tested by these wanton acts of some malevolent force. Perhaps I was just feeling put upon because of an innate selfish trait that most surgeons harbored at least to some extent. I recognized I was probably playing my own "what about me?" victim card because of the disruption Tom's actions had brought to my doorstep. There was always something in cardiac surgery that could bring a large portion of humble pie to the party. It wasn't personal; the gods weren't setting about to inflict all these painful cuts to my psyche, my schedule, or my life. I would rethink that soon.

I met with the operating room director and gave her my version of the two potentially heparin-related profound hypotensive events that had disrupted the schedule and efficiency of the OR. The operating room environment is accustomed to daily disturbances to its charted routines. The exigencies of being at the receiving end of a complex hospital system offering unique and specialized care in a community of gray-haired emigrees from all states and countries prone to freezing weather and the precipitation that accompanied those temperatures was the recipe for daily disruption to any medical entity. We just happened to be the providers of one of the most sought services of our population demographic—cardiac and stroke care. The newly and daily arriving transplants from the northern latitudes brought the health care consequences of their previous living habits. The abundance of sunshine and humidity did not magically cleanse their arteries from a lifetime of high-fat eating and low-exercise living. The smoking habit many of our new arrivals had been addicted to did not relinquish its damage to lungs and heart at the state border. No, we had the apropos moniker of being "God's waiting room" for good reason.

The OR director took in my presentation and information with the steeled confidence of a hardened battlefield commander learning of a break in the defenses along the front. "Let's check those lot numbers of the heparin we used and see if it is elsewhere in the hospital, like the ER and on the patient floors."

"I have already asked Kirk to gather up the vials and check the lot numbers between the two cases and if there is any other of the same lot in the hospital," I replied. "I also asked him to get the Pharmacy director to check their inventory. I'll follow up with him and let you know. This could be a coincidence, but to have two such dramatic reactions on the same day seems a stretch."

As she was nodding in agreement, she got a call from the OR control desk. "Okay, I'll be right there," she said into the phone. Looking at me, she arose from her chair while saying, "The patient in Dr White's room just coded. She was doing a fem-fem bypass."

"I'll go with you to see if she needs a hand," I said as we walked out the door.

The story was like a repeating record. "We gave the heparin, and within a minute it was low to no BP, no response to drugs, and then v fib, and as you see now, we got nothing," said the anesthesiologist as they filled the IV tubing with an assortment of resuscitative drugs.

I spoke to Dr. Sheila White, the attending, as they performed CPR on the elderly patient. "Anything I can do to give you a hand?" I asked her.

"No, Ben, thanks. This guy was adamant about no heroic measures. If we get nowhere from this, we will call it. He's a widower with no children and was adamant about DNR status." I considered that the DNR was probably being somewhat infringed upon with the CPR. Sensing this, Sheila added "I'm going to do the CPR to allow the drugs to circulate, but if no response, I'll call it."

Fifteen minutes later, still in the OR, Sheila, the OR director, and I were discussing the sequence of events with White's patient and the rapid loss of blood pressure following the administration of the heparin. "I've never seen anything like it," stated Sheila, a very experienced vascular surgeon. As I listened to her recount the death spiral, her clinical description certainly seemed to fit the pattern established earlier with the two patients I had been involved with. We concluded that the common denominator was the heparin. I returned to her OR room as they were preparing to move the deceased patient to the morgue and got the empty heparin vials from the trash sack. These clearly needed to be compared with the others that had been used today. I was trying to call Kirk's cell phone to see whether he had gathered up the used vials from the earlier cases. The phone went to voicemail.

I returned to the hallway as Sheila and Bonnie, the OR director, were walking toward Bonnie's office, where she and I had been talking a half hour earlier. "Kirk is not answering his phone. I'm going to check the two ORs where Fry and I were working to see if he got the empty vials. While we get this information together, I think we should find a number or contact person for the FDA. If our suspicions are correct, this could represent a national issue, and I don't think we can afford to not get the ball rolling," I stated. They agreed, and Bonnie started to call the Pharmacy director to get him up to speed and try and track down a contact for the FDA. As she was doing this, I returned to the OR suites to see if I could locate the used vials from Fry's and my case. Both rooms were empty and already spotlessly cleaned. I asked the housekeeper that was just finishing the floor in my room. "Yes, the trash had already been removed," she stated in a heavy Latina accent while she was cleaning. "No, I did not see Senor Larson get anything from the room. The red biohazard trash bags had already been taken to the ground floor for disposal."

Perhaps Kirk got them before the cleaning staff got to the room, or maybe he went down to retrieve them from the trash, I thought. *But why not answer the phone?*

I returned to Bonnie's office to find a police officer there, escorted by one of the hospital security officers. I quickly told Bonnie that I hadn't found the vials as the police officer—in his thirties, I guessed and no longer taking steps to maintain the departmental entrance requirements for weight or fitness—gazed around the room and down the hall to the operating rooms. He was clearly out of his element and kept his hands locked on his hat in front of his somewhat ample waist, as if by moving a hand or touching what was obviously a nonsterile chair or wall, he might somehow contract Ebola or maybe be the cause of the next pandemic. "Dr. Halle," he stated. "The lieutenant wants me to bring you back to the young lady's condo. They have something to show you and have some questions." I suspect my response was what I had witnessed earlier with Kirk's face. Is there a universal fear in being confronted by law enforcement? Does all of society have this innate fear of being accused, even knowing we have done no wrong? What of the citizens of a totalitarian state? If I reacted viscerally like this, how do they deal with authorities where there are no rules, no guardrails of laws to ensure equitable treatment? The image of George Floyd flashed before me. Crazy, I knew, but real, nonetheless.

"I need to see a couple patients before I leave the hospital," I noted. This simple statement seemingly reconfirmed my independence and, at least in this building, a more primal position of my new relationship with the young officer. "Tell your lieutenant I will gladly head over there in about an hour." He seemed happy to accept our new collegial but hierarchal ranking and said he would tell his supervisor I would be coming. I also sensed that this option to escape the alien world of the operating room provided an impetus to get the hell out of there beyond my declaration.

After the officer left, I explained to Bonnie about Tom and Emma's weekend interactions (i.e., altercation) and that when I checked on her yesterday there was evidence of someone having lost a significant amount of blood with no victims around. I asked her to keep this confidential, to which she readily agreed. I then suggested we follow up by phone after she heard from the Pharmacy director and hopefully from someone in the FDA. I had a strong suspicion they would be on us like the locust plague of the 1930s. Were we to be the hospital equivalent of the dust bowl?

The victim of a rapacious governmental carpet bombing of our policies, procedures, manuals, staff education, outcomes, incident reporting, and such? Unfortunately, once they got in the door, it was extremely difficult to get them out—not unlike lice, termites, or *National Lampoon's Christmas Vacation* guests.

ELEVEN

I CHECKED ON the patients along with the physician assistant on call. We determined there were a couple of patients that could be discharged to return the next week for surgery, as one of the partners who was currently at a meeting in Denver would be back at the end of the week. We could catch up on these delayed cases that were exacerbated by the emergencies of today from the heparin and the shortage of a perfusionist. Kirk had said earlier in the day he had a locum coming in for a few days until Emma was ready to return to work, this being stated without my sharing with him that she was currently MIA. I'm not sure why I didn't tell him, but something kept me from sharing. That information seemed important to keep close for now. I sensed a connection between Emma's absence and the issues here in the hospital. What they were was not apparent to me, and I chalked it up to my innately suspicious mind.

I think this suspicious mindset evolved from my encounter and subsequent friendship with Mike, whom I believed to be with the CIA. In medical school, I had traveled on a summer program to Zambia, Africa. It was over all a great experience, and I met some incredible people working in Lusaka, the capital. Most of these were there through non-governmental organizations (NGOs) dedicated to the mission of helping others. During a two-week posting to a small clinic along the Zambezi River, I was startled on the first or second night there to meet a guy who had graduated from USF in Tampa and now ran a "safari camp" centered on the river. He described the tree huts on an island in the river across from the main camp and offered to let me spend a couple nights there at no charge, being as I was there trying to help the locals and, for whatever reason, he took a liking to me. It sounded great, and I quickly accepted the offer. When I got to the camp late one afternoon after traversing the waterway separating the island from the main camp on a large deck boat, I settled in to observe the hippos, crocs, elephants, violet-breasted rollers, red-necked falcons, and myriad other species. The shore across the river was that of Zimbabwe, governed by Robert Mugabe, an autocratic wannabe dictator who unfortunately brought economic ruin to the country through gross mismanagement. While the US had a working relationship with Zimbabwe, my stay on the island outpost brought me into the operational side of what I believed to be the CIA. In the first few hours, I met Mike. He became my new (and now many years later) friend. The amazing Mike Davis—or M. D., as he came to be known—was personable, with an athlete's build. He was about my age, stood at five feet eleven inches, and had blue eyes, curly brown hair, and an infectious laugh. That first afternoon, over a beer, we shared stories of our backgrounds, his Ivy League education at Dartmouth, and his travels before joining his current employer.

In retrospect, it was my life story details that seemed to be discussed: growing up in a small town in Iowa, working both with my father and grandfather in the lumberyard my father owned, as well as on my maternal grandparents' farm. There was pheasant, duck, and deer hunting on weekends, and school athletics year-round. I spoke of life with my younger three siblings and their adult avocations, my college years in South Dakota and summer work doing research through an EPA grant, my marine reserve training, and then medical school in Iowa City. All the while, his self-contributions were of little detail. He stated he worked for a think tank in Washington and was here on the recommendation of a friend to recharge his batteries after a grueling couple of years trying to create predictive models for positive economic interventions from government entities. He clearly had an Ivy League educational mindset I didn't share. I wanted to fall asleep with the mere thought of his work life. His work life, however, proved to be a bit more glamorous than my initial impression. "You want to see some real sick people?" he asked. "I'm going to go over to Zimbabwe tonight to meet a guy who has this economic theory about the financing of health care in the third world. You should come along, and you can explain the actual care being rendered from a physician perspective."

I quickly reminded him I was only a medical student, but the idea of seeing another example of a health care system that was broken appealed to me. That and having another country on my passport. When I stated this, he corrected my misconception regarding the passport. His "guy" was going to meet us on the riverbank across from our island camp. He would then drive to the outskirts of Kariba. As if to justify this entry, he stated there were no passport control sites in the town. He described the place as a significant amalgamation of huts, cinder block structures with metal roofs, and simple lean-tos. "Okay," I agreed, "It sounds like an adventure for my memoir." The river crossing went without a hitch. We could hear the grunting and blowing of water as the hippos broke the surface—an immediate auditory reminder of their presence. Their immense girth posed a danger that could truly ruin a beautiful starlit night. Despite our being in a less-than-coast-guard-certified vessel, the sky was truly breathtaking and kept my gaze upward.

The canopy of the African night is unlike any other. The absence of earthly light contamination disrobes the milky way to express its immense breadth and beauty to those fortunate enough to be gazing from such a vantage. I'm sure the Australian outback and all other outposts of humanity across the globe provide a similar sense of awe and recognition of humankind's miniscule place in the universe. The shooting stars streaming their short laser-like trails and the "twinkling" of those millions not falling give the impression of an intense collection of fireflies suspended over the wandering life-giving liquid highway we were traversing and gave me pause. I knew this water would soon be thundering over the dramatic lips of Victoria Falls in a breathtaking roar of fury and beauty. The ancient native name given this wonder means "the smoke that thunders." The mist at the falls is consistent with a heavy rain shower along its arc of washed stone over a mile in length; the torrent tumbles some 340 feet to the pools below.

A fact I later learned regarding hippos and the night is that hippos kill more natives than just about anything else. These deadly encounters occur near dawn as the villager's head to the rivers for water along narrow trails and run into hippos that have left the water to forage in the safety and coolness of dark, when their sensitive skin is not subjected to the harsh African sun. The impact of a running one-and-a-half-ton leather-encased locomotive on the human body defies description. While hippos are herbivores, they have no compunction about clamping their massive jaws on an object and giving a crushing bite and then tossing it aside. In retrospect, I was glad I was unaware of this as we crossed. The moon was rising and was destined to become a nearly perfect sphere in the next couple hours. Its illumination was now enough to reflect the eyes of the crocs at the river's edge, and the mist flung airborne by the breathing hippos painted an indelible picture in my memory. Crossing a significant body of water in the African night is never a given in a small canoe.

A tall, lean, almost cachectic black man met us and drove us into the outskirts of Kariba, a "resort town" That is principally known for the dam of the same name. This aging hydroelectric dream has fallen on tough times because of inadequate rainfall, poor conservation of the power production, and maintenance. As we drove, I picked up on the conversation between Mike and the driver. It was all about politics and the effort of Mugabe to place his wife in increasingly powerful governmental posts. We pulled up to a simple single-story block structure with a red cross on the front of the building. Mike stated we would go inside and asked me to note whether there were any pieces of newer equipment in sight. "The US and several NGOs have been putting a lot of medical resources and money for the same into this country. We have been unable to ascertain the use of proceeds. We have seen some new equipment at a private clinic in Harare, the capital, but we strongly suspect most of it has been stolen or sold. Some durable medical equipment is probably sitting in a private warehouse somewhere, waiting for the best opportunity or price to move it. This clinic was on some paperwork identifying it as one of the beneficiaries of the monetary largesse. Thus, we—and specifically you—are here unannounced for a brief medical inventory."

We were in and out in twenty minutes. Most of our time was spent trying to communicate with the patients and a "nurse" who seemed nominally in charge, as she was the only professional in the room. The large, open space held maybe thirty beds—fifteen to a side with a central aisle. The beds appeared to predate WWII. The idea of traction for a fractured leg was a bucket filled with water attached to the patient's ankle. The weight of the traction was determined by how closely a family member kept the bucket filled. There were no monitors, cardiac or otherwise, in the entire building, and only a couple of curtains separated a few of the beds. The stench of bloody vomit and rectal discharge was the overpowering odor. The low and continuous moans of many were punctured by the intermittent screams of a girl in labor. This was the white noise of the room. The lighting was that of flickering low-wattage bulbs strung along the ceiling. There were some lanterns on a few tables providing the backup for the inevitable grid failure despite the proximity to the hydroelectric power source. "Mike," I stated as we headed for the Hilux truck we had arrived in, "If they said the money went here, it was being managed by Bernie Madoff"

"Thanks, buddy," he replied. "That was so obvious I could have given that report without you violating the law by your illegal entry into this haven of democratic progress." We returned to our island camp, and Mike sent his report on its way. As we parted the following morning after a late night of alcoholic consumption and my becoming very dubious of Mike's employer story, he handed me a card. It contained his name and a phone number with a DC area code. "Listen, if you ever get to the capital and want a beer, give me a call. Also, since I induced you to become an international felon, please call me if you ever need a hand."

Over the years, on the occasions I made it to DC because of family or meetings, if Mike was in town, we would grab dinner and a drink. He met my wife, Kay, and they, too, hit it off. Mike was everybody's friend. Over time I became more convinced Mike's employer probably had a Langley, Virginia, address. This evidence seemed confirmed after hearing the stories of the places he spent considerable time "working" and while going on a diving trip to Borneo with him. During this "guys' vacation," he disappeared for a few hours during the evenings on our side trips to Kuala Lumpur and Singapore. His stated reason was to check with health administrators for the think tank, but somehow it didn't seem to fit given my profession and him having no qualms in our first encounter of involving me in health-care assessments. At the time, Malaysian-US relations were in the public eye and strained, vis a vis China and its increasing power flexing in the pacific rim. All that said, I knew I could call him if I ever needed to.

TWELVE

I WAS GOING to head to my car when Bonnie texted me and asked that I come by her office again. I walked in to find her seated behind her cluttered desk and facing a suited gentleman. He bordered on portly. His physical dimensions really did a disservice to his natty blue suit and red power tie. His abdominal girth apparently spread some of its excess baggage to his neck. This was evidenced by its diminutive length and layers that fell over the collar of his white shirt, attempting to obscure the knot of red tie facing forward. I wondered for a second whether the red I was seeing was that of the tie or of a constricted neck. He appeared to be in his mid- to late fifties, with salt and pepper hair cut short, as in military heritage. We shook hands as Bonnie introduced him as DEA agent Chuck Harris, responsible for covering Southwest Florida. My first impression was of a bureaucrat on a field trip. The smile seemed genuine enough, but I was unsure whether that was because he was nice or simply happy to be out of the typical administrative warren of responding to redundant, ill-conceived, and IQ-lowering missives from those who have risen to their level of incompetence.

"Happy to meet you Mr. Harris. I must say I thought the FDA might be interested in our possible heparin reactions, I'm surprised the DEA cares," I stated, perhaps somewhat rudely, as I wanted to go back by Emma's condo to see whether she had returned and to call Wyatt, Tommy's' lawyer, to see whether he'd had any communication with her. Additionally, I wasn't sure why

I was a party to a meeting with the DEA, nor, frankly, why he would be in the hospital. His response was cordial despite my brusqueness. "We believe there may be a distribution center of narcotics located here, or at least a connection between this facility and some larger drug rings working the gulf coast of the state." He watched my reaction of honest confusion and frank disbelief before continuing. "We have reasons that I can't elaborate on that somehow medical drugs are being intermingled with illicit ones, primarily fentanyl and heroin. The bad stuff comes in with a shipment of legal stuff and then gets separated. The smack and fentanyl have myriad names on the street: 'crazy one,' 'dance fever,' 'dragon's breath,' 'fire,' and whatever else some poor soul wants to christen it. We have suspected the natural route across the gulf from central America and Mexico has become less utilized, in part due to our interdiction efforts and the unreliability of the contracted mules. That border, while porous, frequently involves disruption at various distances from the actual border from citizen militias in Texas and Arizona. While we don't condone these private endeavors, they seem to have reduced some of the traffic. In addition, the increased funding we have received from congress has allowed us to beef up the coastal presence of our maritime deterrence. We now have some information that the long and minimally controlled Northern US–Canadian border is getting some of the preferential traffic."

"That's all very interesting, but how does that involve us here at the hospital, and being in Florida?" I asked.

"Many of the legal drugs are manufactured out of the US due to tax advantages. These come from Europe, China, and Canada. Those from the latter can be accessed through shipping before or after they cross our border. That said, we believe most of the intermingling occurs north of the border. If after, it is with the collusion of the truck drivers or fleet managers on this side and requires a different route. Now, we readily admit this seems like a long run, but the dollar amounts involved in this can give even the preacher pause to consider a step on the sinful side."

"Again, how does this—and you, particularly—come to our doorstep?" As I was asking this, I wondered where our administrators were for this conversation and why Bonnie and I were the only ones hearing this somewhat fanciful tale. I would have thought people with a lot more juice than I would be the ones to take this briefing.

As if reading my mind, Mr. Harris continued. "We have discussed this with your CEO and given the possible involvement by the Pharmacy Department and the need for absolute confidentiality, we were told you, as the well-respected chief of surgery and a longtime staff member, should be our liaison."

Bonnie then added, "The CEO called me; I told him I thought you were in a much better place to observe and question. I'm considered administration, so my poking around individuals would seem contrived, whereas people come to you daily and confide in you. You are the preacher that wouldn't walk to the sinful side of the aisle, to paraphrase our guest."

I mumbled a thanks and then asked our salesman-suited guest, "Who do you think is involved here?"

"We aren't sure," he replied. "I guess we will leave that to you. But, to help your thinking, we believe it is someone who can manage or interact with the drug shipments and perhaps has spent money that seems out of their expected abilities. Those are the things you might notice or hear about."

My immediate thought flashed to the beachside condo of Emma's. I didn't like this mental journey, and the destination my imagination was propelling me toward was certainly uglier than the sunset vista that her less-than-humble abode afforded her. "So, to be clear, you have not spoken to anyone else in the hospital about this?" I asked.

"No, you two and the CEO are it," he quickly answered.

"What about other hospitals in the state or surgery centers? It would seem like they could be similarly involved," I stated.

"We thought of that and tracked down the wholesalers who provide most of the drugs to the various centers," the DEA agent explained. "While it is a possibility, for the volume of drugs and the ability to minimize the number of people involved, we think the number of the surgery centers and individuals would make it too complex. Remember: we think this requires a major receiving center. Large hospitals fit the needs and can then get the drugs out to the distribution network and the dealers. They want to keep the potential leaks in the system to a minimum."

I took this information but felt dirty simply being on the receiving end of this report. My entire work life had been based on the belief that all the employees that darkened the doorways of hospitals did so with an altruistic sense of purpose. I also recognized that some professionals were motivated as strongly by the almighty dollar. They were in the minority, in my experience, and the farther away you got from those inhabiting the doctors' lounge, the more evident the altruism shone in the hallways and gathering places of nurses, technicians, security, volunteers, and housekeeping. These people weren't getting rich, and job security was never guaranteed in the effort to maintain corporate profitability. No, these were people empowered with a general sense of kindness and gratitude. I did not want to believe that greed was compromising my ORs and hospital. "Okay, I'll ask around and see if anything seems out of the ordinary." I mumbled. "How do I get in touch with you if I see or hear something?"

"Here is my card, and I'm going to send you my contact information. Bonnie—May I call you Bonnie?" She nodded her assent. "Has already given me her and your cell phone numbers. Please call at any time of day if you have questions or suspicions. We need to stop this before it does more damage than it has already." I recalled the consult of the twenty-two-year-old girl I had seen over the weekend. I think he vastly underestimated the damage already done.

We parted with a handshake and my assurance I would be working to find a connection if one existed. I left Bonnie with the same message and headed first to the Pharmacy offices and then to track down Kirk.

THIRTEEN

I FOUND HOWARD Adams, PhD, the thin, bespectacled sixty-year-old, putting some paperwork in a briefcase and preparing to exit his office when I entered. The office was small but seemed to fit nicely around the diminutive man. There was not a piece of paper or hint of clutter or disarray in evidence. A couple of family photos sat on a small side table behind him while the shelves around the room held binders and books with such titles as The *U.S. Pharmacopeia, Dietary Supplements, and A Five-Year Summary of Aminoglycoside Toxicity.* They filled all available space. The arcane nuances of modern-day pharmacy management and the associated relationships to the small compounding companies and the big pharma giants both nationally and internationally required the political skills of Bill Clinton, the imagination of Stephen Hawking, the business acumen of Jeff Bezos, and the financial wizardry of Warren Buffet. The hospital system could easily fall into a black hole of cost (i.e., profit loss) if the Pharmacy Department was not kept reigned in. The constant desire of the physicians to try the next wonder drug, cost be damned, was kept in check only by the artful guidance of its director.

"Howard, good to see you," I said, reaching for his hand. We had served on many committees over the years but didn't socialize or cross paths outside of the hospital, this probably being due to my innate hesitancy to be around most hospital personal off the premises. By and large, I felt them to be primarily focused on their day jobs, and the conversations generally felt contrived.

That's not to say I didn't have good friends from medicine, but those individuals tended to display and be enthusiastic about their outside interests and passions. Perhaps I was a little arrogant and had been accused of such by simply being a heart surgeon. It seemed to me that I spent an inordinate amount of time in the hospital, surrounded by the repetitious "cut from the same mold" sorts of people. When out of the hospital, I wanted a different experience and conversation. Most of my friends constituted a wide range of vocations, ages, and tax brackets. Perhaps Howard would have been one of those, but the opportunity to explore friendship had never presented itself in my recollection. Perhaps he thought differently about missed encounters I didn't know. I guess that like all things in life, perception and perspective are always uniquely a solo asset. We may try to share with others and do on occasion find what we believe to be complete convergence of emotions and thoughts, but even those instances are fleeting. Our neurologic composition and its stored memory experiences are always just ours. Even those moments shared, such as having a child, being in a car accident, seeing a movie, are unique to us individually. They can't be taken from us. Where there is overlap with our spouses, friends, and family, our experiences can only be related to what we share and what they accept from their experiences at the time. All of it is impacted by the environment surrounding us contemporaneously: emotions, weather, level of relaxation, anxiety, and so on. All shared memories are distorted by something in each of us. That is the limitation of humans to see like others. It's always through our eyes and not theirs.

"I see you are heading out, but if you have a couple minutes, I could use your expertise," I stated.

"Sure, I just want to get to my son's baseball game. He's a senior at Canterbury and having a good year at the plate. Hitting around .300 and starting center field," he replied.

"No problem, I'll be quick. I'm wondering about the three patients we had today that seemed to have profound hypotension after the heparin and would not respond to the usual pressors to get the BP back up. I have asked Kirk Larson to gather up the vials, but are you aware of any other instances like this? Has the FDA had any warning notices posted, and did the FDA get called today?" I asked, trying to limit his delay.

"As to your first question, I'm not aware of any reports of similar reactions and have not seen anything come across my desk about it. I did call the FDA, and like you, they want the used vials to get the lot and production numbers. This most likely represents a contaminant of some sort. The FDA response team will be here in the morning and, hopefully, after querying the national reporting database, may have some ideas. I haven't seen Kirk, and I also called the OR desk and left a message for him to get us those used vials. You may or may not be aware Kirk gets his OR drugs shipped directly to him to manage. It was felt that one less middleman between those using the drugs and the distributor would improve efficiency and reduce costs in time and handling. I also left a message for the distribution manager to call me. He was out of the office today, so I expect to hear from him tomorrow. I thought he could also get us the lot numbers that went to Kirk's last few OR orders to see if they differed from the rest of the hospital."

"Thanks, Howard," I responded, "I really appreciate your efforts and the information."

"Oh, one other thing, I told the night Pharmacy manager to get some heparin from Tampa Presbyterian tonight so we can isolate our supply until we have a handle on this. It should be arriving at any minute. Fortunately, the cath lab is quiet, and they are holding the elective stuff until we get the replacement drug on premises and checked in."

"That's great, Howard," I said as he headed for the door. "I know the administration will be grateful for your actions. Go on, get to your son's game. And good luck. I hope the cougars win."

I next walked to the office of Kirk, our chief perfusionist, who seemed to have gotten sidetracked in his assigned mission to get the used heparin vials. Unlike Howard's neatly organized office, Kirk's was reminiscent of Sanibel Island after hurricane Ian. There appeared to be chaos on top of clutter on top of what can only be described as complete absence of order in any sense: open folders, strewn manuals, loose papers, a collection of tubing parts, pump heads, and a variety of tools that could potentially repair them if enough pieces showed up to this dance of disorder. I had been in Kirk's office many times before, and while not "neat," it never rose to this level of carnage. *What happened here?* I wondered. *Is something missing besides the occupant of the room?* That thought was of course somewhat rhetorical because no one would ever know if something were missing.

I scanned the top couple of layers of debris, thinking as an archeologist might about trying to minimize disrupting the upper layers too much to get a look at the depths of the sediment, this being represented by personal evaluations, pump maintenance records, perfusion records of patients, and the like. I was hoping to see something about heparin shipments, dates received, or something similar. I saw no such file or even what might be the remnants of such. I looked around the room a little slower. There were some file folders on the floor, but again nothing that seemed pertinent to the day's issues. There were a few photos on the wall, reflecting a passion for fishing, and in particular walleye fishing. There was Kirk and others, standing in front of a cabin with a stringer of walleye. The caption said, "Fall Lake June 2009." Another showed the same cabin in the background, but this time a mix of northern pike and bass were featured. There was a picture of Kirk and a man I didn't know on what appeared to be a deck, having a beer. The caption said, "Zaverl's July 4th." Kirk had sometimes talked about his love of northern Minnesota, telling fishing stories and tales of treks into the Boundary Waters Canoe Area Wilderness. These were relatable to me, having grown up in northern Iowa and fished frequently in Minnesota. The boundary waters is a huge, preserved wilderness of over a million acres and accessed only by canoe. No power equipment is allowed. The most frequently used jumping off point is out of Ely, Minnesota. As described by Kirk, this is a small town on steroids. They have a large 4th of July parade, and according to Kirk, beer consumption on the street is the norm. He also described the blueberry festival in late July, where every conceivable blueberry-filled or -decorated consumable can be found, as well as hundreds of artisans selling their goods. I had bookmarked Ely in my brain as a vacation destination based on Kirk's glowing reviews. I pushed the vacation thought aside as I tried to understand what happened to Kirk and the empty vials we needed to collect. *Jeez, how come no one will stick around to talk to me?* I was beginning to develop a complex.

FOURTEEN

I STEPPED INTO the early dusk of evening. The western sky, visible from the parking lot of the hospital, was awash in a palate of color. Brush strokes of soft orange, pinks, and violets, reflecting from the base of the clouds, aligned in a daisy chain dance line extending to the horizon. The color and mood soothed me and inspired me to believe some goodness was perhaps in store. Once in the car, I again tried to reach Kirk on my cell with no luck. I then called Tommy's lawyer, Wyatt Slife. He, at least, wasn't avoiding my call, but then he was probably billing Tommy for the time he would spend speaking to me. I suspected at a minimum of $750 an hour, calculated in fifteen-minute-minimum intervals. "Wyatt, it's Ben Halle. I was wondering if you had heard from Tommy or Emma, the girl that was with him when he was arrested? I don't have the contact information for Tommy at his treatment facility, and I can't get a hold of Emma to see how she's doing."

His quick reply was that he had not spoken to Emma and that his secretary had also been trying to reach her. He had, however, spoken to Tommy. "He says these first couple days have been busy with intake evaluations and an initial stay in the observational unit to ensure that he was not going to go through DTs as a consequence of abstinence from the alcohol. He informed me it was mandatory for all new residents, despite his insistence that he was not that heavy of a drinker. He also informed me that he now understands the magnitude of his dependency and the threat it was posing to his life and livelihood."

"Well, that's a huge first step for him to take," I noted, simultaneously thinking he had only eleven more steps to work on.

"Tom also said if I talk to you, to give you the phone number to his residence hall, and asked that you call him sometime," Slife concluded, what was probably a $187 two-minute information exchange.

"I'll do that. Can you text me that number as I'm in my car?" I asked.

"No problem, I'll let you know if I get a hold of Emma or if there is anything else regarding information about the events of the other night for his hearing. The text with the contact info should be to you shortly."

My phone chimed, alerting me to the arrival of the text message. "Got it, thanks, and I'll let you know as well if I speak to Emma," I added as we said good-bye. I then thought that the text was probably a surcharge that got additionally billed. I then wondered how people would respond if all the trades billed for short conversations. I could imagine the lawn service and real estate agent sending bills for phone calls or brief encounters in the yard to ask if perhaps the guy would mow a little shorter. Were we in danger of evolving into snippets of monetized daily activities valued at some arbitrary number and requiring an annual renewal contract to maintain our service expectations with every little thing we did. It left me chagrined to believe I was becoming the prototypical old man Floridian.

I drove by Emma's condo and on a pass through the parking lot noted the crime scene tape remained up as an impenetrable barrier to the neighbors and me. I realized stopping would not gain me any information and headed home. My mental distractions had managed to place the request to speak to the officer in charge by the messenger patrolman completely off the table. One less thing to do today.

A short time later, as darkness settled around us, Kay and I sat on the patio, waiting for the meatloaf she had prepared to cook. The quiet was interrupted by our low conversation and the deep-throated burping of tree frogs. While I sipped on a glass of red wine, my wife enjoyed her go-to of club soda with cranberry juice and a lime on the rocks. I shared the frustrations of my day and related the suspicious heparin reactions, the absence of Emma, the apparent disappearance of Kirk, and the empty vials. I noted I had met the DEA agent but left the assumption to her that it was heparin related. This assumption, while factual, was devoid of the conversation with the agent regarding drug rings and smuggling. I just felt it probably wrong and premature to mention its possible connection to other drugs. Kay is very perceptive and intelligent in addition to her stunning beauty. "DEA and heparin. odd, isn't it?" She noted, looking for my reaction. I maintained my best poker face. We had met in the OR where she was a nurse. Smitten at first sight, I immediately was committed to convince her she should marry me. The blond-haired, blue-eyed beauty with a body that would have drawn the talents of Vermeer, Monet, and da Vinci to abandon their muses. She always seemed to innately understand people and their problems. I frequently teased her that she should be a psychologist. With that insight to people's souls and thinking, she often educated me about others' intents and motives long before they were evident to me. I ignored her question about the oddity of the DEA and heparin, and she remained silent, understanding that I was not yet ready to give all the details. She did, however, take a new tack.

"Listen to what you are saying and what you are not saying. Emma may or may not be living above her means. Kirk disappears, and both have responsibility on some level for the heparin. I know how it works from my time in the OR. They get the drugs necessary for a case, they deliver it to the patients, and they then do an accounting of what's used, and bills are generated. Maybe they don't have issues themselves, but perhaps someone is using them to get substandard drugs into the hospital. Remember that company that was compounding drugs in New England a few years ago? They were violating all sorts of standards for the industry, and patients died. It may well be a source problem of the heparin manufacturer. You guys may simply be the point of the sword, so to speak. Emma may have disappeared to avoid questions about Tommy, and Kirk may have some other rational explanation for his being incommunicado with you. I share your concern for the two of them and the patients. I think at this point you need more information." Her prescience was always disarming.

I wondered, given her deduction that the DEA was concerned about heavier drug traffic through the hospital, what her insightful brain would construct as plausible scenarios. We heard the timer in the kitchen notify us that the meatloaf was done, and our conversation shifted to family issues—fortunately, none of them of major drama. I was only half listening to the rundown of the day my wife and two kids had endured. There was the usual of teenage girl angst from "nobody likes me" to sleepover plans with her friends, and my son's latest desire to play soccer in the English

Premier League. If only he were faster and had better ball skills—two impediments he didn't yet acknowledge.

As Kay was updating me, I kept returning to the absence of two people and evidence of some violence associated with one of them. If they didn't appear tomorrow, I would give my old buddy Mike, in DC, a call. He also seemed to have a second sense about people and their actions. Perhaps he could give me some guidance. I also made a mental note to call Tommy in the next twenty-four hours to see how he was doing, thinking perhaps he could point me in the right direction as to where we might find Emma. I returned to the present as she arose from the lawn chair and said dinner was ready. We had meatloaf, a mixture of beef, pork, a few vegetables, and breadcrumbs. This seemed to represent and summarize my understanding of the events swirling around me.

FIFTEEN

THE SUN WAS just cracking the darkness of the eastern horizon as I headed for the hospital, the glowing orb bringing its hazy edge above the junction of the far reaches of the everglades and the placid night sky. The cloudless drape of waning darkness always gave me an emotional jump start. The brief commune I spent on such mornings allowed me mentally to prepare and go through the steps of the planned surgical procedures of the day. I never wanted to take for granted the responsibility placed upon me as a surgeon, and I had found over the years that the best way to avoid catastrophes was to plan responses to them before I faced them. I had performed thousands of cardiac operations but still understood that even the most routine and frequently done cases held the potential to turn into life-and-death struggles. While the outcome did sometimes get determined by sheer luck, it more often was the consequence of an experienced and practiced decision tree and team. The experience, real or gained through preprocedural thinking and planning, gave the patient and the surgeon the best chance for success. To paraphrase General Eisenhower, no plan survives first contact with the enemy. It's the contingency planning and preparation that saves the day, and these have bailed me out more than once. I like to think I've carried this into my regular life but, I readily admit, not nearly to the same degree as in the OR. Several of my life decisions and consequences bear witness to this failure on my part.

After rounding on the patients, I directed the physician assistant on the floor as to my desires regarding some discharges, lab orders, and patients coming out of the ICU. The patient I had that crashed from the possible heparin issue would be remaining in the ICU for, it was hoped, just another few days. His renal function had declined from the shock and prolonged time on the heart-lung machine. I anticipated it was temporary, but it was concerning. Kidney failure to the point of requiring dialysis as an intervention was associated with a significant increase in the risk of death. I headed for the OR. I was met by Bonnie, who stated we were again shorthanded from the perfusion staff and that the cases between me and Bob, my partner, owing to the needed coverage of the catheterization lab by a perfusionist, would need to have staggered starts. We talked about the order and the most efficient way to complete the schedule. While not ideal, it seemed reasonable, and I calculated I would get done around seven if there were no hiccups. As I headed to get scrubbed, she informed me no one had heard from Kirk this morning. I asked her to call the sheriff for a welfare check, as Kirk was widowed and lived alone. I then gave her the sheriff's cell phone number he had given me after I had operated on his elderly mother. "Please explain I'm in surgery or would have called myself. And please assure him you won't share his number," I asked of her.

"I will," she stated. "Also, just so you know, we are using heparin we got from Tampa. Since Kirk isn't available, I asked Pharmacy to get in some more for us to replace the stuff borrowed from them and get us enough to carry on until we have sorted out the issues."

"Okay. When I'm done with this coronary, I'll go back to Kirk's office to see if I can find anything that might help sort this out. I don't suppose any of the empty heparin vials have appeared?"

"None yet," she responded as she headed down the hall.

The three-vessel bypass with a piece of the saphenous vein from the leg for two of the grafts and the internal mammary artery mobilized from the chest wall went smoothly, with no untoward reactions to the heparin that was administered. I was out of the room in a little over two hours to allow Bob to get on bypass with his patient and our shared perfusionist. Then I would return to take on a valve repair and replacement. Bob was a very good surgeon, but speed in the OR was not one of his attributes, and thus I knew I had a couple hours to be out of the OR.

I returned to Kirk's office and in a much more organized fashion tried to sort through the mess, which remained unchanged from the day before. I first tried to collect any files related to heparin. There were four different folders labeled as such. One was a collection of articles regarding the drug, its usual dosing for the patients getting cardiac surgery, the use of "activated clotting times" to monitor its blood-thinning effect, and how to address "heparin resistance" in certain patients in whom the thinning effect seemed blunted. There were also articles on the alternatives to heparin in those patients identified as having a heparin allergy. Another file was from the Pharmacy Department, outlining the current preferred vendors for the drugs used during cardiac surgery. Another folder contained shipping receipts that had been signed for by Kirk to accept the drugs. The final folder contained a spreadsheet of weekly and monthly drug volume utilized and ordered. I looked at this a little closer, as I knew our cardiac case volume and thought I may have misunderstood his system, as our actual case volume was significantly less than the numbers on the spreadsheet. And when I pulled out the folder of receipts and it matched his case volume list rather than the actual volume, I knew it to be. Kirk was ordering and receiving significantly more drug products than we were using. This realization caught me off guard. There had to be some logical explanation; I just wasn't seeing it.

I looked through the remaining folders and papers strewn about his desk, chairs, and available floor space. Some were technical manuals regarding the pumps, their maintenance, and their parts. Another was of time sheets and vacation requests for the perfusionist. There were a couple on fishing tackle, seasons of different species, and Minnesota species limits. There was a folder on recommended fishing guides into the Boundary Waters Canoe Area and suggested equipment. This folder also contained a few more pictures with Kirk and various fish, some on a stringer, some lying on a deck, some being held aloft to capture the moment. In a couple of the pictures was an Asian-appearing man of about forty. I didn't recognize him as a local I had met. This meant nothing, but I wondered who Kirk knew well enough to have spent fishing vacations with him. *Somebody in the hospital will know*, I thought. The other repetitive theme was Minnesota. I needed to ask around about his ties there, and maybe who the guy in the picture was that obviously shared important time with Kirk.

SIXTEEN

I FOUND HOWARD in his office and once again was struck by the sense of supreme order in all things surrounding him. I tried to imagine his household with a teenage baseball-playing son in residence. If the kid was like every other boy of that age that I knew, there had to be some raging internal conflict Howard would grapple with every time he was in the kid's room. There is a unique odor of the adolescent male, particularly the athlete. It's somewhere between musk, aging locker room, compost pile, and cheap aftershave. The general nesting area of the teenager is best described as a warren of discarded clothes, unmade bed, and, if a family pet is around, the ever-present napping creature secure in the knowledge no predator would be foolish enough to explore the fabric-hardened redoubt. For the first time, I noted a diploma on the wall from McGill University, which is considered by some as the Harvard of Canada.

"I didn't know you went to McGill. That's a great school but a little unusual for a US high school grad," I noted.

"Growing up in New Jersey, I had exposure to a lot of cultures," he replied, "and I thought I would continue that in a foreign country, albeit one that is about as American as America is. Montreal was a good place to gain the 'foreign' element and to grow. I made some great friends from abroad. Roughly a third of the students were foreigners. I found the Asian kids to be the most fascinating, probably because of the difference in about every measurable and objective parameter. That said, I became good friends with a few and appreciate the relationships to this day."

"I had no idea of your cultured worldliness," I noted, chuckling.

"Well, it's not something I advertise, I guess. I've made a couple vacation trips to visit my friends and am always grateful for the experience," he added.

"How did your son's game turn out?" I asked.

"We won with a walk-off double, bottom of the seventh. My kid played well. Went two out of four at the plate and made a great throw in from center to get a runner at third." He spoke with obvious pride. "I suspect we will see that team again in the playoffs in a couple of weeks."

"That's great," I replied. "Reliving our youth vicariously through our kids is one of the perks of parenthood. It gets tricky, though, when the parents try to insert their imagined life into and onto the kid. My dad tended toward that side of the spectrum. It ended hard for him when I quit playing football in college to concentrate on premed. He let me know I disappointed him, as my athletic success was somehow the way he defined his own as a parent. I've taken great pains to not be my father, as many a child has. Tell your son congratulations on the win and the season. I know he doesn't know me, but I'm always excited to hear of the athletic and academic successes in the community.

"The reason for my visit, if you have a minute, was to ask you to walk me through the process of how we get the heparin, mannitol, and solumedrol for our pump cases."

"Sure, no problem. The system is about to change, but we are not yet converted hospital wide," he replied. "For the drugs you use every day, historically Kirk, or whoever headed the perfusion group, would place an order to our distributors for the needed drug and would manage the invoice statement and present it to me for payments. The management of inventory was left to him. We are in the process of getting everything loaded onto a central server that notifies the distributor of an order and then gets a reply that acknowledges the order and, when shipped, gives the tracking information to us so we know when to expect it. The whole system should be operational in a couple months. Though one would think the lessons that could be learned from the Amazon model would have made this a straightforward deal."

"What if our distributor doesn't have the needed stock? Does the new system know where our other potential vendors are, and are they on the system as well?" I inquired.

"The biggest distributors will eventually be on the 'grid,' so to speak. But that is down the road as we work through the government regulations, as some of the drugs we might need are limited to certain conditions that require health information disclosure—which is protected, as you know. Trying to get the protection built into the system is more complex than the writers of the HIPAA legislation envisioned. Similarly, the smaller generic drug manufacturers are going to be delayed in the onboarding by us."

"Given the supply chain shortages we keep hearing about as the cause of some of our medicine scarcity, it would seem the current system will need to remain in place to allow you and Kirk to source what we need," I noted.

"Yeah, I think the automated system is going to be a process. The hospital IT department is very anal about security and control of access into the system. The hoops outside companies need to jump through and the indemnification the hospital wants to have in place to prevent data leaks and, God forbid, a complete hijack, with introduction of some ransomware that could truly cripple the entire place, is keeping those guys up at night. I don't mind the old way of talking to whom I'm doing business with." He gave a subtle smile.

"Do you and Kirk check with each other about orders, timing, et cetera?" I inquired.

"Usually not. He can get what he has ordered from the delivery dock or here in the central pharmacy storage area if he is not there to claim it on arrival," he explained. "I don't look at his orders, and I doubt he has any interest in the stuff ordered from my office." He then added, "I'm not sure what to make of the heparin issue of the other day. I personally checked the received heparin we had, and it all seemed to square up with Kirk's orders and lots that were shown to have been shipped. I'm inclined to think it a unique coincidence, but I'll be showing our stuff to the FDA agent today."

"For the common drugs, like heparin, do you use more than one source?" I asked.

"We have relationships with quite a few distributors and belong to a purchasing group for many of the drugs we use. If we, or really the distributors, are having trouble sourcing drugs, we start making calls to avoid the shortage as best we can."

"Do you ever deal with the manufacturers directly to avoid the middleman?" I wondered out loud.

"As a rule," he responded in a professorial tone, "the manufacturers don't want to deal with us individually, as the time and number of accounts for the unique drug needed would be an additional headache for them and the integration of all the different IT groups. If they are a small compounding facility, the expense would obviously impact the production and sales cost. So, for us to deal directly with the manufacturer holds no benefit to them."

I was getting the impression my questions were beginning to annoy the head of Pharmacy. "Thanks, Howard, I learned a lot today. I hope your son continues to do well with his baseball career." I left the department feeling as though I was missing something in the explanation I had just heard and thought this was probably a result of my not asking the right questions, but there was something making me feel unsettled. I really needed to talk with Kirk directly and was afraid that his vanishing act was becoming more incriminating by the hour.

SEVENTEEN

THE COMING SUNSET of the night before had brought with it not just cooler air but also the immutable table saw buzz of mosquitoes. Emma had no idea that this variation of waterboarding could be as effective as the standard version for breaking the spirit of someone. Between the buzzing and the biting, the anticipation and reality of the constant itching made sleep a fantasy as real as her being the next person to climb Mount Everest. She had used the scratchy blanket as a very poor rendition of a mosquito net. It had kept some of the little bastards out, but she needed to leave space to breathe, and thus the port of entry where nothing was rejected was open to her larger self.

They had delivered a plate with a sandwich of dried turkey that could well have been left over from Thanksgiving a year ago. There was a glass of water. Apparently they didn't have certification for the well water brought up by the handled pump in the cabin. *If what it discharges is worse than the tinted stuff in the glass, yikes,* she thought. The offered water had some discoloration approaching a rust color, and a taste to match. They made her hand her pee bucket out, and she heard a splash on the ground outside as it was quickly returned to her. Thank God for her inclination toward constipation, as thinking of the butt-meeting-bucket humiliation only brought more despair. She had noted the sandwich delivery guy appeared Asian in his facial features, and she had heard muffled voices a couple times during the night, as if a couple of them were strolling the area after sunset. Also, around sunset she had heard the lonely-sounding call of what must have been a loon, though to be fair she had never heard one before, so this was conjecture on her part. The minor delight to her was that another bird answered to the first. *At least they aren't alone*, she noted, trying not to shed a tear upon this realization. She again, for the thousandth time, tried to figure out what she had done to get to this place and, at the same time and the same number, what she or someone else was going to do to get her out of it. She thought she had heard a motorboat a few hours ago, but she'd had only the sounds of the forest to keep her company since. Those sounds of chirping, occasional screeching, insect wings, and the rustling branches of pines and leafed trees—aspen or birch, she thought—were her companions for now. She had not heard human voices for a few hours now. She mentally created a checklist of things to note and be aware of during the next encounter: footsteps, heavy or light; the smell, height, and attitude of her captors. She decided to try to engage them. All these things, she felt, could play a role in her survival.

EIGHTEEN

AFTER LEAVING HOWARD and returning to the OR to complete my last case, I knew I needed to run this by someone I trusted. I was not yet convinced Chuck Harris, the representative of the DEA, was in my circle of trust. As I was scrubbing in, I mentally made my list of to-do things: talk with Tommy, call my buddy Mike for worldly guidance, and continue my search for Kirk. I also wondered why we had not heard anything about Emma. This snake ball had no beginning or end in sight, and unraveling it seemed to carry the potential for a lot of pain for someone.

The valve repair required only a supportive ring on the annulus, or base, of the mitral valve, and the replacement of the aortic valve with an Edwards Inspiris Resilia bioprosthetic went smoothly. There were no issues with the heparin, and I was completing the case earlier than I had anticipated. I exited the OR and spoke to the family. I thought I would have some time to work on my list after seeing a couple of consults that had been prescreened by one of the physician assistants and decide as to the best course of their treatment. The options being surgery now or in the future for the first consult. After reviewing the patient's echocardiogram and heart catheterization and examining him, we decided to have him discharged, discontinue his smoking, and see me in my office in two weeks. If he had stopped his pack-a-day smoking habit, we would get him on the schedule. The other patient was in her mid-eighties and had symptoms of aortic stenosis, shortness of breath with minimal exertion, a fainting episode, and occasional chest discomfort. She needed a new aortic valve. Again, after looking at her echo and heart catheterization films, and following the exam, I laid out the plan to obtain a CT scan of her heart that would give us the size of the valve to be replaced as well as to check on the size and presence of plaque in her arteries from the femoral artery in her groin to the carotid arteries in her neck. This study would need to be delayed a couple of days because of her marginal kidney function. We did not want to give her more contrast to allow us to image those structures so soon after her heart catheterization and risk injuring her kidneys. I explained this to her. I then described our recommendation to replace her valve using a catheter with the new valve attached. We would advance the device from her groin. The transcatheter aortic valve replacement (TAVR) would be done with some mild sedation and local anesthesia. I thought she would probably go home a day or two after the procedure. She was literally beaming upon hearing this. The physician assistant stated, as we left the room, that he wished we could do all the cases that way. It was frankly easier on all concerned when we did these—not that there weren't risks involved, as I noted. "The avoidance of prolonged ICU stays, and the short hospitalization frees beds and resources for other patients with critical needs," I stated. Being a big proponent of this, my endorsement was easily aroused.

It was nearing six o'clock as I headed for one more look in Kirk's office and to ask around among his office mates whether they had any information that might give a clue as to his whereabouts. Unfortunately, there was no one around his office to speak to. I once again looked at the papers and records that were strewn about like yard leaves on a windy fall day. There had been no organizational effort here since my last visit. I again looked at his pictures of fish and fishing companions. I thought I would share this with DEA agent Chuck Harris. I again noted the same cabin in several of the photos and the Asian-appearing gentleman with Kirk in another. There were pamphlets from outfitters, all based in the town of Ely. This seemed to have the connection to Kirk and his companion. I took the pamphlets, though I was unsure as to what to do with them in my quest to locate our perfusionist. I was unsure where Kirk lived but thought that if Bonnie had gotten the sheriff to do a welfare check, there probably wasn't much danger in looking at his place if I could get in. I called Bonnie's office, and fortunately she was still there finishing some reports.

"I'm assuming you got the sheriff to do a welfare check on Kirk, but I thought I would stop by and check it out if you have his address?" I stated.

"The deputy called me back and said everything looked fine" was her quick reply. "Here is his address if you really want to stop by there." She gave me the address, and I thanked her and disconnected. I phoned Kay and let her know I would be home in about forty-five minutes.

Kirk lived in a small, non-gated older development of houses built in the seventies and eighties. The trees lining the street were mature oaks, some fruit trees, as well as fifty- to seventy-five-foot-tall jacarandas and their purple-blue flowers capturing the angled rays of the western sun and giving a warm hue to the streets below. While the trees were indeed beautiful and provided a refreshing break from the monotonous palm-treed landscape of every other Florida development of the last twenty years, the variety and individuality of the homes also made the statement: "We are from somewhere else." Those residing here were not likely newly transplanted northerners seeking sunshine, no state income tax, and a golf cart to minimize the steps to and from their cookie-cutter home, duplex, or condo. Those items closely associated with the actionable trifecta of golf, a nap, and cocktails. Thus fulfilling their idea of heaven's waiting room. Kirk's house was a one-story with a two-car garage to the right front and a walkway from the driveway going left to the front door. I walked to the door, rang the doorbell, and knocked, with no response. I was walking around the back to seek another potential entry point when my phone rang. I looked at the screen and saw that it was Kirk. "Doc, I saw you on my Ring doorbell," he explained. This immediately answered the question about his earthly presence but not yet his whereabouts.

"Kirk," I nearly shouted. "Are you okay? Where are you?" I got out before he said anything else.

"Doc, I'm okay, and I know this looks bad, but I'm trying to get it straightened out," he gushed.

"Listen, tell me where you are so I can help," I answered.

"I don't think you would be safe if I told you. The cops were at my house, I saw, so I know things aren't good."

"The cops were here checking on you at my request," I explained. "The real issue is simply if the heparin is bad and how do we isolate it!" I barked. I could feel my frustration rising and did not want to lose this conversation to egos or irrational fear.

"Doc, I think we are in the middle of some bad shit, and I'm not sure if or how I got us there," he noted with some trembling to his voice.

"Do you know where Emma is?" I asked.

"No, but I'm looking for her now," he replied.

"I appreciate that, and I want to help you. Tell me where you are, and I'll come give you a hand." I tried to speak calmly.

"Doc, you take care of the patients. I'm out of state, so you won't be able help," he stated emphatically.

"Out of state where? At least tell me where you are looking for her? This is bullshit, Kirk. I can help you clear this up." My exasperation-laced voice captured my rising anger at his secretive obstinance.

"I don't want to say just in case they are somehow tracking this call or me directly. I know my way around the area where I think Emma may be. Listen, we need to end this call. I will try to call you again." And the phone went dead.

I slowly retreated to my car and replayed the conversation over in my mind. He'd said something that struck me about "knowing" his way around the area and being out of state. I wanted to get into his house to check whether he was truly not there, but I felt that with his watching the home security system, I would look foolish—and frankly criminal, to be honest. Was he being truthful, or was this a ploy to distract me and allow him more time to flee whatever problem he was mixed up in? Was this the issue the DEA wanted to get into? It seemed very likely that Kirk's contribution to all of this was getting more involved, whether he understood that or not. If Kirk was afraid of someone tracking him, it appeared as if the unseen forces I was dancing with should be considered with caution. This again reminded me of the blood in Emma's condo. I wasn't prepared to speak to the police, as I had no real information and didn't feel that a call to Mr. Harris of the

DEA needed to be made tonight. I needed to consider all I knew and try to bring some order to my thinking. The best way to do that would be to speak to friends and have a glass of wine. I slowly pulled out of Kirk's driveway as I asked Siri to call the number Wyatt Slife had given me for Tommy at Hazelton.

NINETEEN

I LISTENED AND considered the situation of my day and dilemma as the miracle marriage of miniaturization and societal demands delivered its most ubiquitous life enhancement to me and most of the "advanced" world—the connectivity from virtually every location, including my car, to a friend located nearly fifteen hundred miles away, around the corner or around the world. This immediacy of access had altered my work and social life just as it did for every other sod who allowed himself or herself to be made hostage to work, scams, or social media feeds. I could converse and receive a to-do list from my spouse. I could affect the management of patients in real time. I could check on the activities and location of my kids. It was like being omnipresent without the need for being present. The obvious consequence was that many of us simply never reverted to actually being present. I really struggled not to slide down that slippery slope of the "typical" surgical persona: never home, never available to family, never on time. The cell phone could help me or push me further toward absenteeism. I needed to maintain my vigilance to the present. My reverie was jolted to the present by a pleasant male voice that aborted the electronic noise of ringing. "This is Jim, can I help you?" it asked, as if the sole purpose of this voice was to make me content.

"Yes, Jim, this is Ben Halle; I was hoping to speak with Dr. Tom Moore. Is he available?" I replied, wanting to somehow make this voice understand how it was indeed helping my day.

"I think he is in the common room. I'll go take a look." This gracious response seemed to exude the concept of a higher power or spiritual core one would expect from a Buddhist monk—an attitude of service rather than the one of indulgence or indolence that was so frequently expressed in the interactions commonly confronting us in our daily lives. I realized I was making a large and minimally supported assumption regarding this unseen and unknown "Jim," but the feeling was strong and immediate. It felt good to believe in good.

The next voice was that of Tommy. "Ben, how are you, man? I want to apologize for letting my problems spill onto your lap. I know you have had to deal with the crap I left behind, and I really appreciate it. How is the workload getting dealt with? Are the guys stepping up to the plate to help with the consults, office spillover, and cases?" He got all this out before I could say hi.

"Tommy, it's okay," I quickly interjected. "We are all getting the work done, and more importantly we are committed to doing whatever we can to support you. We agreed to pay you as if you were here, and we will try to protect your vacation days—if not all, most—depending on how long you need to be there or not working full-time when you get back." "Thanks buddy, "was his emotion filled reply. "So, tell me about the place and if I can do anything to make it easier." I earnestly asked.

"The trip up was fine. Someone met me as I exited the door of the plane. I guess they have a pass from TSA to meet new arrivals to the program, thus short-circuiting any thought of a quick drink at a concourse bar before entering the program. I give them credit for the effort, because as I got off the plane and contemplated a life without drinking, the desire to have a couple for old times' sake was strong. I could mentally taste the smooth vodka on ice all the way from Florida. When you check in, they go through a long intake process; but even if you state you haven't had a drink in days, they place you in sort of an infirmary. You share a bathroom with a similar new arrival also seeking health and sobriety. Fortunately, neither of us displayed evidence of developing DTs. Though to be honest, I did have weird dreams about being trapped in an OR room, being forced to operate with some kitchen utensils, and having all the partners watching through some glass viewing gallery. You guys would laugh because my hand was trembling, and the patient was awake and yelling at me, and lights were strobing in the room Now, I intellectually know this was about giving up control of my life and being powerless over alcohol. This, I have learned, is the first step of the twelve-step program. However, it was so real it could have been the hallucinations of DTs. I did not want to share that, fearing I would spend more days in the infirmary setting. I would think what we do would be some comfort in such a place but no, not as the patient.

They moved me to a section of all male professionals. They are very cognizant of the ability and vulnerability of opposite genders to seek solace in all the wrong places. Thus, our only setting interacting with the women is at the speaker events in the auditorium or in occasional larger group sessions. We haven't had any of those yet, but the agenda is very tightly scripted, so you know well in advance of your commitments. The place is like a college campus. We have a cafeteria and a library—albeit somewhat heavy in the science and psychology of addiction, but with other genres as well. There is a meditation room, a pool, and a full gym. We start early in the day and meet with counselors, psychologists, family therapists, et cetera. Every hour is accounted for. I like the regimen. I don't have to be responsible for other lives. I just show up and do the work on myself. In my short time here, I am beginning to gain insight as to the choices I made in life and why a good many of them were bad. I have a long road ahead, but I am looking to the day of self-clarity and control. This journey also brings me to another favor. Would you consider coming up here to meet with the psychologist and describe me from your perspective? I realize Sue would be a more logical choice, but her codependency and frankly selfish interests would not be helpful. They said they would accommodate your timeline and travel limitations. Again, I know it's a huge ask, but I want to get healthy, and God knows I need help." As he spoke, he intoned the sincerest voice I had ever heard him use. Perhaps the water they were drinking contained a supplement that promoted humble interactions with others. I hoped they sold it in the gift store if there was one. I wanted to spike the drinks of a few people I knew.

"Yeah, I'll come Tom. You had me at the college campus description," I quipped. "I'm joking; I want you to be healthy and happy. We will all be the better for it. Listen, have you heard from Emma?"

"No, why?" was his quick response.

"Well, she has been MIA for a few days now. I don't know if she thought the issue with you and the courts was too much or if there is something else going on. Did she ever say anything to you about maybe having some other issues to deal with or problems at work?" I asked.

"Not that I recall. She said that sometimes Kirk seemed distracted or perhaps secretive. She said if he was on the phone and one of the other perfusionists or she walked in, he would quickly mumble a good-bye and get off the phone. She figured it was some woman since he was widowed and didn't want to let them into his personal life. Emma then said this secrecy had gotten more obvious over the last couple months. She suspected this 'relationship' with a mystery woman was deepening. I don't know if that might be involved in Emma being absent. I must tell you, Ben, I'm getting some bad feelings as I talk." The sincerity remained in his voice, but perhaps the "goodness" it carried was slightly tarnished by our conversation and its implications.

"Tommy, I will call you in the next couple days to let you know when I can get up there," I said as I pulled down my street in the waning suffused light of the western sun. It's display of muted colors dampened by my mood as much as the thunderheads filling the void of the vacated space of the horizon-bound orb. What would the next day bring as that life-affirming sphere approached us from the opposite direction? I hoped for good but, like a bad kid at Christmas, was prepared for the worst.

TWENTY

KAY JOINED ME as I had a glass of wine, and she tried to normalize the current world I was residing in. She caught me up on the day she and the kids had had. The lives of a nine-year-old boy and his somewhat bossy, ten-year-old sister was consumed by video games, war games, and soccer with brief periods of mutual displeasure followed immediately by loving gestures. If only adults could be so openly vulnerable. It was nice to know that some aspects of my life were proceeding on that road most of the world calls "Straight and Narrow Lane." I didn't have much to offer but expressed once again my gratitude for her to being able to keep the kids and our life organized around the unpredictability I brought through the door. I told her of Tommy's description of rehab, and we both concurred it was the best and only option for him to maintain a license and a life of purpose.

When we got to the phone call from Kirk, she listened intently and asked whether I knew where he might be "looking around." I wasn't sure but given the DEA concerns and the "being out of state" comment, I wondered out loud whether it wasn't a northern state bordering Canada. This conjecture then lost its strength as we both contemplated the possibility of the longest international border in the world. As we talked, I googled the border and was informed it stretched over fifty-five hundred miles, with only one hundred land border crossings. It left a lot of open space to move about. Without more information from Kirk, I wouldn't know where to tell someone to look for him. Something about setting Kirk up for a manhunt seemed premature and a little like a betrayal.

Kay then asked whether I had spoken to my buddy Mike Davis, the somewhat mysterious but always helpful friend I'd met in Africa so many years ago. Her question reminded me that calling Mike had been on my list but somehow got pushed aside by the day's details. "Kay, once again you are acting as my brain. I was going to call him on the way home but got distracted by the conversations with Kirk and Tommy. It gets proven daily that you are not just another pretty face. Thanks for the reminder."

Her quick reply was "If I have to prove it to you, I'm not just a pretty face, I think I'm failing."

"Sweetheart," I replied, "You don't have to prove anything to me or anybody else for that matter. Having you as my partner and confidant is all I want, and the rest of the world can go eff themselves if they think you are anything but the hottest, smartest, kindest person on earth."

"Okay, lover boy, you might be lying, but that kind of talk could get you laid tonight. Why don't you call Mike, and I'll finish up dinner, and then later …" She coyly smiled, walking toward the kitchen. God, that sort of talk was hot, distracting, and totally appreciated by me. She really was incredible.

Mike picked up on the first ring. "My favorite doctor! How are you?" was his greeting. This was followed by "And Kay and the kids, how are they?"

"We are all good and miss you, *mi amigo*" was my reply. "How are you doing? Are you in the States?"

"All good here. Still single, though I have been seeing this gorgeous lady who works at State. She seems to think more of me than is justified," he answered with a note of pride in his voice.

"That's great," I said, "but obviously this poor girl needs some serious therapy if she is consorting with the likes of you. If you really like her, please let me speak to her about an intervention before she hits the love speed bump that is Mike Davis. I hope you have a fund established to assist all the discarded Davis lovers that can no longer function in civil society as a consequence of their succumbing to the wily charms of my good friend."

Kay stuck her head out and yelled to Mike after catching a bit of our conversation, "Mike, you'd better get that girl down here so I can make sure she understands what she has gotten herself into."

Hearing this, Mike responded, "I'm not sure she is ready for the brutal interrogation I know you two would deliver. Guantanamo would look like a picnic compared to the sort of intense soul-bearing forces you can muster. If you would promise to be extra nice and say what a wonderful guy I am, I could see a visit to Florida soon."

"What?" I exclaimed. "You want us to endorse what you are selling to this woman? You must be really smitten. This is serious—unless you think bringing her here will provide an opportunity for her to 'get lost' in the everglades, thus removing your impending guilt for breaking yet another heart along the DC beltway," I laughed.

"While I do appreciate your historical perspective and concern for the broken hearts that don't require your services, I do think I like this girl a lot," he said calmly with a chuckle.

"Okay, I promise if we get to meet her, we will be on our best behavior and lie if that's what it takes to promote your honorable intentions toward all women. Now this bit of subterfuge, if you will, is going to cost you a small favor," I said, thinking, *no it isn't*. I would do anything for my buddy, but it made the ask easier.

"Sounds like a deal. What do you need, Ben?" he quickly offered.

"Mike, we have a little problem here, and it seems like the issue is perhaps much larger and more complicated than most involved realize. If you have a few minutes, I will give you the highlights and then pick your brain a little."

"You have my undivided attention," he replied.

"Great" was my answer. "Here it is in a nutshell. We believe we have gotten some contaminated heparin, the anticlotting drug used for heart and vascular surgery and to treat deep vein thrombosis, or DVT. The drug we received induces profound shock, and therefore one of our patients has died. The other two could have easily also joined the line at the pearly gates, but we somehow got them through the acute event. We had a visit from a DEA agent named Chuck Harris, who seems to believe we are also getting illicit drugs coming from the north in addition to the bad heparin. The money in heparin is peanuts comparatively, so I'm not sure a northern smuggling cartel makes sense. He or his bosses seem to believe this northern route is just being created and trialed to determine the practicality of this as a true moneymaker. We have seen an uptick in ODs and drug-use issues in the last year. We seem to have lost our innocence from the drug business despite the average age of the county being over fifty and the neighboring county sixty. Age now is no longer a predictor of drug innocence, since many of these elderly have had surgery for back issues, and joints repaired and replaced. The wide use of pain meds pre- and post-procedure have captured a whole new cohort of addicted individuals.

Sorry to get into the weeds a little, but the failure of the medical establishment to use common sense and not be coerced into thinking any pain reflects poor care just pisses me off. You had patients pointing to a particular face ranging from smiling to neutral to sad, then tearful, to express their pain level. This then became a marker for the quality of care. If anyone had pain, the nurse, the unit, and the hospital were dinged by the accrediting agencies. These agencies, frankly, were incentivized to find problems. Hospitals were coerced into justifying the cost to be a part of such agencies and pay for the right to be told, rather arbitrarily, you were good, as opposed to comparing themselves to national benchmarks of quality established through data. No, the subjective marker of pain became a measured vital sign. This opened the floodgates to the overprescribing of pain meds and the subsequent social disaster virtually every community is facing all these years later. When you've got Grandma looking through Grandpa's meds to get the monkey off her back because she had a knee replacement a year ago, you've created a whole different-looking addict than the public wants to admit." I ended my soliloquy here. "I guess I'm asking if you have any buddies in the DEA that could give you a little more information about this possible narcotic traffic in addition to our heparin issue. I really want to figure out this heparin problem, and as quickly as possible. If we can determine the contaminants and the source, we can prevent disastrous outcomes here and elsewhere."

"I didn't mention that two of our perfusionists are missing. The cops aren't really looking too hard for our chief perfusionist, Kirk, as they don't yet seem to realize he isn't around. The other is a female, Emma Ridley. I think she was abducted and potentially murdered, but other than blood in her condo and an inability to contact her, I've nothing to go on. When I spoke to Kirk earlier tonight, he acted as if he knew she was alive and was looking for her. He would give me no information about any whys, how's, or where's. So, with this bit of background, do you think you could check it out for me?" I asked, not trying to sound desperate or pleading, though that's exactly what I was doing.

"Listen, Ben, I am in awe of what you do every day; the time and commitment you have given to help others makes the rest of us look like the poachers of life. We complain about lines in the grocery store or having to wait for an Amazon delivery or, frankly, waiting to see a doc who is so overwhelmed by patient volumes and paperwork that he could easily take the role of Howard Beale in the movie *Network* and say, 'I'm mad as hell, and I'm not going to take this anymore.' I'm not only going to check with the DEA, but I might have a couple other doors to bang on. This is not a favor you are asking; it's requesting governmental assistance in areas where you perhaps lack expertise. I, my friend, can play in the areas you need looking into. Give me a day or two and I'll get back to you. Oh, and the girl's name is Joyce when you meet her."

"You do this for me, and I can get back to a normal level of crazy. I'll tell Joyce you walk on water, save pets from trees, and do the dishes. You will sound like me, but not as good looking," I teased.

"All right, tell Kay she shouldn't put up with your juvenile mind. I'll call you as soon as I have something," he said, and we bade one another good-bye. My juvenile, prurient mind led me to the kitchen for dinner and what I hoped would be dessert served in the bedroom.

TWENTY-ONE

EMMA AWOKE ACHING from the aging bruises and those added to her back and sides from the three-inch mattress, whose created intention was to fake one into believing he or she was going to be treated to sleep. The ground outside the cabin had to be less deforming than the wannabe mattress in the cabin. She had received a couple meals a day, in the morning and late afternoon. She suspected evening fires were being avoided to minimize drawing attention, but this was only a guess. She had only heard the voices of two men, and that was all that she had seen during the last thirty-six hours. She could not recall the numbers from her condo and nothing of the trip to wherever this was. The mosquitos didn't seem as bad this morning with the sun up, but dusk and dawn were the hell she expected God had created for the wayward souls destroying the environment. The blanket was still her only protection. She would gladly pay an exorbitant amount of money for some DEET-containing repellent. Her goal today was to ask to get outside, even if shackled, and to see the sky and perhaps beg for some repellent; she smelled it on her captors, so she knew they had some. She doubted they would let her out, but nothing is gained if you aren't trying. If they did let her out, even for just a few minutes, she could perhaps get a clue as to her location.

Her stomach was cramping a little, what her constipation had been holding back would soon be delivered to the bucket in her "jail." She did not want to attract the flies with the mosquitos; that would be insult to injury, and her mental state may well cave to the cacophony of buzzing twenty-four hours a day. She was pretty sure the flies didn't take a break when the sun was up like the mosquitos, especially if there was a bucket of crap to get their attention.

She heard the steps of one of the men approach the door. "Step back" was the command in clear English—perhaps with a Canadian accent, as he said he was "aboot" to enter. Emma stepped back, and the roughly six-foot muscular man stepped in. His slight smile seemed to hide a malevolent subtleness that accentuated her stomach cramps, but this iteration of cramps, she knew, was not related to constipation. He seemed to fix his eyes on her chest, and a thinly veiled threat seemed to come closer to the surface. Her filthy T-shirt and jeans, with the enhancement of several days of odor clinging to every thread, could not have been appealing to any sane male, or so she thought. His slightly Asian eyes were dark and capped by thick eyebrows. Those hairy features almost created shadows below which the eyes sought refuge from whatever the retinas wanted to avoid. *Probably things like giggling children or flowers in a forest*, Emma thought. She smelled the repellent that the atmosphere within the confined space now carried. This quickly brought her voice to her lips as he continued to stare at her breasts. Apparently, these were not things those eyebrows would protect the retinas from.

"If you have a latrine, could you take me there? I need to crap, and the bucket in here won't handle it," she said as authoritatively as possible, hoping this might place him in a somewhat subservient role. Then again, playing a poor damsel in distress might have been the better way to go. His leering fixation on her boobs pushed her to the authoritative mode. No pun intended, she thought, *It was a crap shoot.*

He stared at her for what seemed like an eternity and then spoke. "I'll walk you oot there, but if you try to run, scream, fight, or do anything other than walk oot there, take your shit, and walk back, I will kill you." To emphasize the point, he pulled a large handgun from the back of his trousers. His free hand set a tray holding a bottle of water, a bag of nuts, and a couple of power bars down.

Not a lot, but better than nothing, she thought. Feeling emboldened by her success, in the best authoritarian voice she could muster, she said, "I appreciate that, and I understand. I have no desire to get killed. But equally, I have no desire to be eaten alive by the mosquitos. Could you let me use a little of your repellent?" He again took his time, as if the decision would alter the balance of world power or at least allow him to stare at her chest a while longer. "I'll think aboot it while you take your crap."

They exited the hut, Emma in front and completely convinced the gun-toting Canadian-sounding jerk was staring at her ass the entire time. He directed her to stay on a narrow path that was well worn, and the adjacent ground to one side sloped gently down for about twenty-five to thirty feet, then went on to a marshy bog that looked to be filled with scrub trees and moss. This was no doubt the home to millions of her mosquito tormentors. It was reminiscent of the Everglades but with a much more moderate temperature and a third of the humidity. Back about fifty feet or more from the front of marsh were some stunted spruce trees maybe twenty to thirty feet in height. To the other side of the path was a large stand of pines and what appeared to be aspen, birch, or both. She was unsure. The thought of it being among aspen brought to her the random factoid about aspen stands all being of one organism. She recognized the complete lunacy of such thinking, given her current circumstance. Still, she hoped it was aspen. Community of any kind now felt important, even if it was composed of trees. While the woods were relatively thick, the slender breaks between the trees afforded her a glimpse, farther down a gentle slope, of water perhaps a quarter to a half mile in the distance. The shimmering reflections created the daytime equivalent of twinkling stars on earth. She strained to hear or see any boat traffic. The only thing she noted was a sense of hope brought about by the water's presence between the trees. Maybe she could talk this pervert into taking her down there to wash up. She would have to think about it.

The outhouse was about one hundred feet down the path. Beyond that another twenty-five to thirty yards was a small log cabin with a porch facing east, toward the lake she had seen. The cabin was rustic in appearance from the outside. Lying next to it was a canoe. She could not see any motor vehicle on the gravel space that seemed to extend toward the far side of the structure. There appeared to be a gravel road beyond the cabin into the forest. This she took in quickly as Mr. Pervert was directing her into the outhouse with the admonition to "be quick aboot your business." There was no need to encourage her, as the smell and flies within the one-hole crap station was enough to make a freight train take a gravel road. Fortunately, there was some toilet paper that perhaps had come from the same trees as the logs for the cabin. To say it was abrasive would be like saying Moby Dick was just a fish.

After completing her task, she quickly buttoned her pants and exited the throne room. Mr. Pervert waited with gun in hand. "How about the repellent?" she said, swatting at her neck, arms, and face in a vicious cycle of constant repetition. Perhaps it was the slapping and itching that gave her companion pause, more likely the opportunity to ogle her body a little longer. He directed her toward the cabin. It was quiet inside, but then her escort shouted, "Hey, throw me the mosquito repellent." Without comment, the screen door opened, and another man, perhaps an inch or two taller than Mr. Eyebrows, with the same ebony-dark hair, cut marine-boot-camp close, stepped out with the can of repellent. In contrast to the closely clipped hair, he sported a short, well-trimmed beard, its blackness equaling the caterpillar canopy shielding the retinas of captor number one. He eyed Emma, this look being more akin to sizing up an adversary than looking at a potential sexual conquest. It was silent, intent, and the piercing black eyes left no doubt as to the violence he might inflict if he desired to or was required to. His frame was taut, and the muscles, while well defined, were not of the gym-rat density but more like those of an extremely fit endurance athlete.

Emma felt more threatened by this marathon man than her current pathway companion. She tried to look past him into the cabin, wondering whether there were more of these assholes around. There was no movement she could detect, and the knowledge that she was being stared at made for only a chance glimpse. He tossed her the can of repellent with his right hand. She caught it without fumbling and quickly applied it to every square inch of her body as ravenously as a man dying of thirst gulps lifesaving water.

"Take it easy, we doon't have any more," Marathon man snarled. "Get her back in the hut. We doon't want her to feel like this is a vacation," he continued in the voice of command. Hierarchy recognized and established.

While trying to delay this moment, Emma quickly asked, "Why am I here, and where am I, exactly?"

The menacing short reply of marathon man was simply "Get going."

In returning to her confinement, Emma noted that the current path stopped at the door to her shed of a jail. Beyond the structure, the forest was set back ten to fifteen yards, then its dense underbrush created a wall of green and brown with the constant rustle of the branches and leaves of aspen, giving a comforting cadence to her steps. The kiss of air moving across her bruised cheek somehow imparted solace to her, much like the touch of a mother's fingers to a child. Her dining cuisine of power bars awaited her. *It could perhaps be worse*, she thought, remembering the implied threat of the ass-watching man trailing her.

TWENTY-TWO

THE EARLY-MORNING QUOTIDIAN cadence was normal, and frankly I was feeling quite chipper, having been the beneficiary of Kay sharing my desires for "dessert" the night before, and having temporarily compartmentalized the issues swirling around me. This compartmentalization was shattered when I opened the door to find an atmosphere-induced mental gloom, dropped in the form of a rare but heavy gray summertime fog. It obscured the commonly recognizable physical attributes of our home, yard, and neighborhood. It provided the perfect backdrop to the reengaged murkiness and cluttered chaos that was my thinking. I couldn't realistically believe either Kirk or Emma was involved in drug smuggling, I was worried that the hospital and they were somehow victims. Yet the degree to which some unknown party put this all into motion did not seem realistic.

I drove slowly toward the hospital, splitting the leaden wet air with my car. This separated the smokey, gauzy mist only momentarily, as the auto displaced the blanket where it was and then the space was quickly refilled by the moving, mercurial air vacated by the passing machine. The slow pace only heightened my anxiety as to the etiology of the drug mystery and the ultimate disposition of Tommy's dilemma. It was hard to believe the gods would create such bedlam randomly. But then again, what mortal among us could discern the paths placed before us, the ultimate prize not collected until the final day—or, as some have so succinctly stated, "until the fat lady sings"?

— TOXIC INTENT —

I arrived but a few minutes later than usual and tried to keep a smile on my face. I did not want to provide any more fodder for concern to the staff, who seemed to be now engaged in feeding the omnipresent gossip tree that inhabits every office. The hospital environment, however, seemed to take gossip and rumor propagation to levels that rivaled those of the greatest of internet influencers: Bigfoot was being treated in the ER. The staff was having wages cut 75 percent so the CEO could receive a bonus. The staff was going to receive 75 percent pay raises because the CEO was donating his salary. The stories changed by the hour, and the credibility never seemed to waver. No, I thought it best, as a rule, to not in any way try to confirm or deny the stories. The more outlandish the tale, the greater the consumption—a microcosm of today's distorted news outlets.

I was making rounds and commenting on the progress of our two heparin disasters when my phone chimed. Looking at the screen, I saw it came from Bonnie's office. "Ben are you in the building?" was the question from the director.

"Yeah, making rounds and then headed to the OR for my first case. What's up?" I answered.

"The cardiac cases are being cancelled for now. Come on down to the office when you are done with rounds so, we can discuss a plan."

Now, this was not going to in any way dampen the noise in the rumor mill, nor make life any easier for those of us trying to assuage the patients and families over delays. "I'll be down in twenty," I stated.

I completed seeing the last in-house patient and then visited with a patient in need of a thoracic aneurysm repair, the aortic artery diameter having increased from 4.3 centimeters to 5.5 centimeters in the period of one year. The physician assistant had already seen the gentleman and briefly described the probability of addressing the aneurysm in the descending aorta with a stent graft. I explained that the aorta was supplying blood to his spinal cord and the abdominal organs, as well as that the lower extremities had developed a bulge—or, to the southern crackers, a "pup on a tire." This he understood, and that we would be placing the stent inside of the aorta to relieve the pressure from the blood that was contributing to the aorta expanding further. He would need follow-up scans over the coming years as some of the aneurysms continued to enlarge, but at a much slower rate. The stent would be placed through his femoral arteries. The risk was quite low but potentially could result in paralysis on rare occasions, along with the potential for strokes, kidney failure, organ failure from clots, and plaque within the aorta being dislodged and blocking arteries downstream. The patient, undeterred, took it all in and asked when we could proceed. Given my yet unclarified information about the cases being cancelled, I said we would get back to him later that morning, but we may discharge him and have him return for the elective procedure. I then headed to Bonnie's office and girded for more bad news. To steel myself, and as much out of habit as anything, I stooped in the surgeon's lounge to grab a cup of coffee. Hospital coffee now came in two iterations, the first being from the tried-and-true commercial Bunn coffee maker with built-in water source and a warming element on top to keep one of the two decanters always at the ready. These babies can pump out gallons of hot coffee hourly, taste be damned. It was this technology that fueled the hospital industrial complex that every OR nurse, doctor administrator, or trainee grew up with until this century. The art of consuming the equivalent of 10W-40 oil ranging from lukewarm to scalding is simply another of the undefined and unspoken talents acquired during surgical training or being around those being surgically trained. The introduction of the single-cup selectable drink from a menu of latte, hot chocolate, americano, espresso, and tea seems to have somehow softened the edge to those willing to wield a scalpel and violate the integrity of the human body. I believe the societal implications have been to lessen the narcissistic rantings of those of us that expressed a God complex in and out of the OR. It could be that the diminution of unadulterated caffeine is the equivalent of antibiotics for the infected surgical soul. It could also be that society just doesn't tolerate the assholes among us like they used to. My theories aside, I suspected the hospital administrators would, at some point, recognize the cost associated with trying to tame the unruly with gourmet coffees. In their cost-benefit analysis, choosing to provide the sludge as they had through the decades and removing the refined cappuccino machines would be a no-brainer. It was okay with me. I was old-school. I got my very hot coffee, added just a little cancer-inducing white powder that sat in bulk canisters next to the coffee, and headed for the office.

Bonnie's greeting was succinct and forceful. "Ben, the FDA is concerned with our heparin supply and, as importantly, how it got contaminated. They are convinced it was a bad lot but are still trying to genetically decode it." This made sense because heparin is generally sourced from slaughtered pig intestines or from the lung tissue of cattle. The world's primary source of the drug is China. The number of slaughtered pigs annually in that country is said to be roughly two per individual. Given the population, you are looking at six to seven hundred million hogs. This volume alone, if they were all cleared for medical use (whatever that required), could support the pharmaceutical needs worldwide. The use of bovine, or cow-derived, heparin as an alternative source is smaller but is still a significant factor in the medication production elsewhere. The bovine heparin was not used in our hospital.

Bonnie continued: "They also have reports of a couple of similar cases in the country. The distributors or middlemen are apparently different, and they haven't yet identified the manufacturer. I guess they are meeting some resistance from the Chinese. There appear to be interpretive differences in the definition of quality standards between the countries. I know, shocking, right? The bottom line is that the FDA's interpretation mandates we stop using our heparin until this gets sorted. Emergent cases that must get done will be allowed. Urgent cases get transferred out, and the elective cases wait. I know this is a pain for all of us, especially the patients, but that is where we are. The feds say we were lucky because at a couple of other places they lost several patients to this."

"Do you or they have any idea how long this moratorium will be in place?" I asked.

"I tried to get them to at least guess, but like all bureaucrats, they don't want to say something that comes back to bite them. Given the urgency and implications for patients, international trade, and politics, I suspect they are going to double-check their findings before any definitive statement is made. The problem, as I understand it, will be to determine if the issue is related to the animal itself, the manufacturer, or something interacting with the drug postproduction and occurring anywhere along the delivery chain. I can only imagine the limited influence the US statutes and protocols have in China. I would assume there is more than one manufacturing facility, and who knows how many different slaughtering plants provide the tissues for processing. The quality control variables between those steps are probably not what we would tolerate in the States. I've never been to China, but my provincial opinion is that they don't require the same regulatory rigor we do."

I considered this for a minute, realizing I had not given much thought as to the source of our drugs and simply assumed the FDA controlled all aspects of the system. It was a sobering thought to realize that the susceptibility of the health care system, or at least a critical part of it, was at best loosely under the auspices of those we trusted to ensure safety and quality to the drugs and procedures we performed. I felt as if we had somehow traveled back in time to the days prior to Upton Sinclair's *The Jungle*. The consequences of that book had been the impetus for Theodore Roosevelt to sign a couple of laws in 1906, one setting forth regulations for the meat packing plants and slaughterhouses, the other creating rules for labeling food and drugs. It was the beginning of our current regulatory environment. For better or worse, we needed to protect ourselves from the greed and lack of moral clarity many members of the corporate world exhibited. I, like Bonnie, had not traveled to China, but I also shared her mental image of a poorly regulated medical enterprise. I had traveled and operated in enough third-world places to know necessity and greed usually trumped protocol.

"Given this new world integration and the impact it now has in biting us in the ass, I'm guessing we will be shut down the rest of this week. Don't you?" I stated rather churlishly, though that was not how I wanted to sound.

Bonnie's response of "Yeah, I don't see them getting this cleared up by the weekend. We are going to need to source some heparin and whatever else we were getting through that distributor. We should be all right for emergencies, but word of this has reached all the heart centers, and rightfully they are trying to maintain their supplies in case these spread beyond what we currently know. I've got a meeting with Howard Adams shortly to go through a list of possible vendors to Pharmacy."

"Okay, I'll see about discharging those we can and arranging transfers for the urgent cases that should get done in the next forty-eight to seventy-two hours," I replied, and headed for the door.

TWENTY-THREE

I HAD COMPLETED the discharge and transfer rounds and returned to my office to see if everything there was under control. Our office staff had been doing well keeping Tommy's patients in the system and dividing them among the partners to manage. There seemed to be no issues currently as I sat at my desk trying to read some information on heparin. I contemplated how to best keep the balls in the air when I remembered Tom's request that I come to Minnesota to provide some firsthand knowledge as to his history and personality, since I had known him from internship all those years and wives ago. I really was conflicted as to the timing, given what was going on, but then realized that with cardiac surgery being put on hold, I would be underutilized here. The burden of emergency heart surgery had significantly declined with the advent of coronary stents and the sometimes cowboy approach by a few of our cardiologists. To tackle any lesion, no matter the complexity nor the number of vessels involved, was not a factor a couple of those colleagues considered when performing a heart catheterization. It was quite hypocritical given their insistence, with the advent of coronary bypass years earlier, that randomized double-blind studies be completed before they would allow their patients to go under the knife. Yet when the knife, so to speak, got to their hands, the requirement for such scientific rigor fell by the wayside. "When you have a hammer, everything looks like a nail" was the adage that came to mind. This thinking led me to the conclusion that circumstances now allowed me the opportunity to go north to try and be a friend.

I called the number for Hazelton once again and was not surprised to hear the voice of kindness and civility on the other end. It wasn't the same person whom I had spoken to previously, but the tone and inviting comfort were similar. I wondered whether Tommy would sound as neighborly to those he addressed in the future. I wondered whether the process of self-awareness and giving oneself over to a higher power as part of the twelve-step program created this soothing personality in all comers. I thought, *If that is true, maybe this twelve-step thing should be a part of our educational process.* Well, separation of church and state probably restricted that, but still there was potentially a huge gain if civility were the mindset let loose upon our society. It was nice to imagine political discussions revolving around the issues and proposals without the rhetoric of debasement. Imagine people actually listening to other opinions and debating them with facts that are agreed upon as facts, not distortion. It was at this point that my reverie broke, as I knew I was thinking like a crazy person, and Tommy's voice returned me to the moment. I tried to listen to see if he had yet captured the "grace" of self but could not detect it in his greeting.

"Ben, buddy, how are you today? I hope all is well with you guys. Again, I'm so sorry to have put this burden on you all. I'm going to make it up to you, I promise."

Maybe there was a hint of greater good creeping into my friend's pores. I hoped so, as it would be great to be around such positive feelings regularly. "Tommy, I think I'm going to be able to get up there this week. We are in a surgery pause currently."

"Surgery pause? What's that about?" he asked.

"We have a supply chain issue with the heparin, so to be safe, we are pausing, all non-emergent cases." I answered. "I'll get a flight out tomorrow and then meet you Thursday. If you can check with your 'therapist' or whoever, I will be glad to speak to them. Do you need me to bring you anything?"

"Ben, that sounds great. If you could get some of my workout stuff from Sue, I would appreciate it. I want to use the gym and hate to buy all new again" was his reply.

"Everything going okay?" I asked.

"To be honest, it's tough being truthful about yourself. I mean, really honest. To try and answer why some things triggered me to drink, what I thought of my childhood, why my marriages failed. Just a lot of baggage I've been carrying around that I was basically ignoring or ignorant of—not sure which."

"Tommy, I'm proud of you for facing this. I can only imagine what it takes to confront yourself in front of others. Keep it up. I'll swing by your place and get your stuff. If you could let Sue know I'll be by, I would appreciate it. If there is a hang-up in my getting up there, I will let you know. If you get a time from your therapist or counselor for me to meet them, could you leave me a message at home or call me directly? I'll see you Thursday."

"Will do, and looking forward to seeing you, my friend," he said before we hung up.

After a few moments, I headed to Howard Adams's office. I wanted to know who selected the drug distributors and whether there had been changes in the contracts for producers; the use of pig versus cow, or bovine, sources; or even if we had a say in the product origin. As I approached his office, the door swung open.

The normally organized countenance of his demeanor seemed to have been subject to an emotional gale, leaving him suspicious in attitude and glum in appearance. I interpreted this as fallout from the equivalent of a body cavity search by the combined meaty-handed feds of the DEA and FDA. I suspect that if I had seen his backside, it would have displayed recent chew marks. Howard tried to compose his features as he approached me, and I greeted him. "Howard, you look like shit. I'm sorry you are being put under the microscope, but hopefully this will be short-lived."

"Thanks, this is not fun. I'm trying to find, collate, and copy in triplicate the last three years of drug orders, invoices, vendor agreements, payment histories, contracts, and signed receipts of deliveries. I'm an organized sort of guy, but some of this paper is not in my files; it's scattered in the system between Legal, Shipping and Receiving, the satellite pharmacies, and God knows where else."

I felt sorry for the guy, and I could sense the stress he was feeling and displaying. Being buttoned up so tight in day-to-day living and working does not provide one with a pass on the human frailties of fear and failure. I wanted to put my arm around him and say it would be all right but thought he might lose it altogether if I somehow invaded his physical space. "Howard, again, I really am sorry for this. We will get it straightened out. I know you are being put through the wringer, and the good news is that we could have had a lot more deaths. Do you mind if, for my own edification, I ask you a couple of questions?"

"No, that's fine, Ben. I appreciate your kindness. What do you need?" he asked.

"Well, given this unpredictable response to a drug we use daily, I wanted to know what control we had over its procurement. Do we specify porcine or bovine origination? Do we get stuff from various distributors? Also, do you recall if there was a change in manufacturer by labeling or something? I know the contracts are handled by Legal and there is a buying consortium with several hospitals, but I have no idea if the drugs fall into that joint purchasing group"

"We don't select the manufacturer of origin; that is done through the distributors. We do have them sign a 'best practices' agreement saying the tissues are harvested in a humane fashion and that the manufacturers abide by the applicable rules and regs of the FDA. Frankly, we, as the end user, have no idea if there is compliance with those agreements, and I suspect the FDA doesn't have as much in China as they want or need. We aren't sending anyone to China to monitor them that I know of. I doubt they would allow outsiders enough access to accurately evaluate them if we were. We have not specified the type of heparin, either porcine or bovine, because while there is bovine heparin, it has been banned from most countries since the 1990s over concern for mad cow disease, or bovine spongiform encephalopathy, the theory being it would afflict humans if treated with a product from an infected cow. To my knowledge, there have been no changes in the providers or distributors, or in the contracts. But, again, Legal manages the contracts. Though I think I would have known or been told if there were changes. I also believe that with the events going on, if there had been a change, somebody would have said something."

"Howard, who is our distributor, and where are they located?" I asked.

He paused a little, as if telling me would violate some nondisclosure agreement. "It's Capitol Medical Supply out of Minneapolis," he slowly offered. "I've been dealing with them for several years now. They are very responsive to us."

"Do they know what's going on?" I asked. "Yeah, I and the feds have all called them, and to their knowledge there has been no change."

"Okay, I guess that's something. I appreciate your help, Howard, and If I can do anything for you, please let me know," I concluded.

"I will," he said as he headed down the hall in perhaps a more distraught mood than before he saw me.

TWENTY-FOUR

WITH THE DAY yet young and the ever-present high humidity wetting my clothes and mood, I walked to my car, planning to go home and pick up my Glock and go to the range for a little practice, defuse my frustrations, and allow Tommy time to contact Sue, letting her know I would be dropping by to pick up his requested clothes. I had asked my secretary to make my flight reservations to Minneapolis and, as I was unsure as to how long I would stay to visit with Tommy, leave my return open. Being a frequent flyer for meetings, lectures, and case proctoring, as well as having set up the monthly conversion of my American Express bills to miles though my Delta rewards program, seemed to have induced the airline to treat me well with upgrades and a concierge service that was available if needed. These perks were greatly appreciated by this traveler.

When I got home, I spoke to Kay about my short day and the commitment I made to visit with Tommy and his therapist or counselor. She was glad I could go and provide him some needed support. She was adamant there was nothing pressing on our calendar, as I had already confirmed myself. Kay, with some justification, felt that she was the only one in the household who understood the commitments to sporting practices, school events, and social obligations we had. I had been making a real effort to improve my own accountability by keeping a calendar as well. But she still was not a believer in my prowess toward this aspect of our life. I would just have to keep working on progress and not perfection.

I said my secretary should be calling with my flight details shortly, and with that my phone did its musical role of interrupter much like a three-year-old demanding a parent's attention.

The caller ID was an unknown, but I answered anyway—again, old habits. The advantage of caller ID was lost on this indiscriminate consumer. "Ben, it's Mike. I wanted to get back to you as soon as I could."

"I have to say, Mike, either you are really good or there is something published in the DEA daily, if such a thing exists," I replied.

"Well, let's go with the former, and I'll not mention the huge favor someone owed me," he noted, chuckling. "It appears there have been concerns over substandard medicines being bought and distributed by those inclined to inflate their profit margins. Some of these same distributors are also thought to be importing, through less-than-recognized ports of entry, other drugs that are then placed in the public domain—that is, on the street—by old-fashioned dealers. In this instance, the middleman looks to be a reputable business, and the cash proceeds are easily washed through the business. You mentioned your friend the northern fisherman, and that he said he was out of state. I'm wondering if it might be Minnesota?"

"Why Minnesota?" I asked.

"My DEA buddy said he was just returning from there after looking for some connection to a few medical companies. According to him, the twin cities are a real hub of medical device and related companies. My buddy apparently was unsuccessful in finding anything, but he intended to keep looking in the area." he concluded.

"Mike," I said, "that would seem to fit with what I heard. It seems the heparin distributor is a company called Capitol Medical Supply, out of Minneapolis. I'm going up to see my partner at the Hazelton-Betty Ford clinic in a place called Center City, Minnesota. It is not far from Minneapolis. I might swing buy and look around."

"Ben, why don't you let me do that, or I'll put my buddy onto them to run down? I know you want to get to the bottom of this, but you aren't exactly in marine shape to kick down doors, kick ass, and take names," he noted. "I'm afraid the door would break your foot, you'd miss their ass entirely, and you'd forget the names," he added at my expense.

"Wow, that bit of unvarnished truth wasn't necessary. I see my looking around more as an intellectual exploration of the business and its players. I would pretend to be a hospital representative, which technically I am as chief of surgery. I would ask for their manufacturing sources, delivery method—be it in-house trucking or contracted out—the cost currently, and the frequency of changes. You know, the kick-the-tires-and-not-the-doors sort of inspection."

"I still think you should have me with you as your associate. If these guys are dealing serious drugs, they won't hesitate to see some calamitous events come your way. And by 'calamitous' I'm thinking car accident or suicide by whatever is the route du jour, though given their ready accessibility to lethal drugs, my money is in a narcotic overdose. I don't want Kay to raise your two kids with some douchebag car salesman or something. Though, on second thought, she could finally get a good-looking mate, profession aside. Seriously, if you are going to go anywhere near there, I'm coming. I have some time off—and I have some federal IDs, so that may get us through a door you can't kick or open on your own."

"All right, uncle. You can bring your ugly mug and cute Fed IDs, and we will ask a few questions. I'm planning on going tomorrow, but I don't have my flight stuff yet. I'll have my secretary call you with my flights, and we can talk tonight or in the a.m." I reluctantly agreed. I then quickly added, "If this goes really fast, we might want to try a few hours of walleye fishing since we are going to be in the land of ten thousand lakes—or some such number."

"Okay, I'll plan on showing you how the big boys do it. You probably aren't aware, but I have been pronounced in the past as the walleye slayer—the most feared fisherman to ever toss a Rapala Jigging Rap," he gloated.

"I'm sure you have to use jigs so you don't get those dainty hands dirty with leeches or minnows," I retorted. This had become our routine—a regular Laurel-and-Hardy act typically witnessed by only us. It made me feel good to have Mike counted as such a good friend. I realized that he and Tommy were my two closest confidants, and I would be lost without either of them. "You will be glad to know I'm headed to the range today just to be sure I maintain my shooting superiority over my dainty-handed self-proclaimed fish slayer friend who shall remain nameless," I chided.

"My God, you are such a poor, delusional sod. How do you get through the days without me? I suspect Kay lays out your clothes every morning and constantly tells you what a stud you are. I'm going to need to remind her that these lies are frowned upon in the final judgment." He laughed at his own joke.

"All right, enough of your incessant effort to somehow make you feel like you have anything to offer humanity. I need to get going. I'll talk to you later," I said, concluding the conversation.

Kay had caught a good bit of the conversation and asked if what she had heard about potential danger was real. I tried to reassure her it was testosterone-fueled banter. She knew the way Mike talked. She said she did and that that's what worried her. When he wasn't competing with me in some stupid bet or one-upmanship, he was a serious guy. She held no illusions Mike hadn't been in some difficult situations and got there from his patriotic sense of duty mixed with a moral standard of right and wrong. While she conceded I, too, had that same moral standard, my impetus was to help someone and not beat him or her. "I don't want the two of you to goad yourself into some stupid competition that leads to pain or worse for either or both of you. You aren't that active marine anymore." She spoke with some concern showing in her eyes and on her brow. That was the second time that day I was reminded I wasn't what I once was. This quickly led my thinking to the Toby Keith lyric "I'm not as good as I once was, but I'm as good once as I ever was." I appreciated the different context of the song, but I felt I still had enough of whatever was needed to be a friend and subtle seeker of the truth. "Honey, I don't think there is any way in hell this trip will be more dangerous than driving on the highway or maybe a fishhook in a finger."

"Well, just remember those fingers and hands are needed by your patients," she stated, trying to sound a little more lighthearted. I loved her for the effort and quickly kissed her as I headed for the gun safe to retrieve my gun and change into some shorts and a T-shirt.

TWENTY-FIVE

I HAD TRADED my original Glock 17 for the newest fifth generation model a few months prior. It felt the same, as I continued to use the standard seventeen-round magazine. The gun was only eight inches in length and, unloaded, weighed under twenty-five ounces. Like all handguns, it was not made for distance, the effective range being roughly fifty to fifty-five yards. I had added a red dot sight that improved my accuracy beyond ten yards and felt that the rough-textured grip was an improvement made on an earlier generation. I wasn't shooting competitively, but they had flared the mag well for rapid magazine exchange, and if I were using this in covert situations, I'm sure I would have also appreciated the nonreflective black coating to a greater extent. That said, it was a cool firearm, and I enjoyed the discipline of trying to improve my accuracy with it. I had a concealed carry permit but felt that somehow having the gun on my person was an invitation to a confrontation I didn't want.

I was here to repair the damaged bodies, not to do the damage. I accepted my contradictory views on owning and shooting a gun but felt that armed civilians in malls, in movie theaters, or on the roads led to many a confrontation that need not occur. The statistics on armed good Samaritan interventions leading to good outcomes versus accidental injury to self or others was won by the latter. We all want to think we can maintain our cool and only shoot the bad guy if the time arises. The reality of the adrenaline rush, chaotic scene, and poor accuracy to begin with creates a scenario of innocent John and Judy Doe getting shot by someone—that good Samaritan trying to hit somebody else entirely or, in a millisecond, misidentifying them as foe as opposed to friend. People trained in such scenarios sometimes make mistakes. The repetitive training our SWAT, Delta, and SEAL teams and hostage rescue personnel all continually repeat is designed to avoid making mistakes in the fog of combat. The good citizens should focus on being aware of what is in their environment. It would be much more practical. I had these thoughts every time I went out to shoot.

    I placed the gun in its travel case and headed for the door. It was at this time that my secretary phoned and thus delayed my exit a few more minutes, giving me my travel itinerary and a hotel reservation near Tommy's treatment center to spend the night. I thanked her and asked that she text the information to Mike, whose number she had. I noted I would arrive in Minneapolis around 11:00 a.m. I asked her to get the address and phone number for Capitol Medical Supply and send that to me and Mike as well. I also asked her to reserve a rental car at the airport. While I could have performed these tasks as well today, I was usually tied up in surgery or meetings throughout the day, so my trusted secretary, who also doubled on occasion as a babysitter to the kids, gladly assumed the tasks of getting me where I needed to be, and on time. I had not yet tackled this professional portion of my calendar work as I was trying to do with the family commitments. To be honest, my short, grandmotherly secretary tried to keep me headed toward progress on that front as well. She knew perfection would never be achieved there. The good news was that she was okay with simply trying to help me get better. I believe she did it because it was needed, appreciated, and generally not too taxing.

In addition, I gave her a great Christmas bonus and gift every year. Yes, I was okay with inducements for those making the effort. A true capitalist.

I got to the range and found the parking lot with plenty of spaces. I recognized it was midday Wednesday, and thus most of the patrons were at their jobs. I greeted the clerk as I paid for some targets and 9mm ammo. I was assigned a shooting lane and donned my new Walker's Razor Slim Electronic earmuffs. These are a godsend. They are comfortable and allow you to talk with others or hear commands on the range while blocking the loud reports of gunfire. I got to my lane, attached a target to the track system, and deployed it at ten yards. I shot ten rounds, retrieved the target, and marked my hits. I deployed it to twenty yards, repeated, and then did the same at thirty yards. I was shooting great and believed I was finally mastering my red dot sight. I was sorry Mike wasn't there so I could get one up on him, though from experience I knew he was just as likely to outshoot me on any given day—frequently by wide margins. I went through the sequence several more times and scored within a few points of each round at each distance. I was getting consistent—a good sign.

I stopped by Tommy's place, and Sue met me at the door. She was pleasant in a rather superficial manner, as if I were to blame for her marital estrangement, her husband's alcohol abuse, and now the need for treatment. She handed me a gym bag of his stuff and was about to close the door when she added, "Ben, I think you know Tommy better than anybody, and that's cool. I wish you would have told me this was part of the package I was getting in marriage."

I wanted to say I barely knew her before they eloped and that anyone who had been around him closely for more than a couple of weeks probably would have felt there could be issues. Instead, I answered, "Sue, you are right, I probably know Tom as well as anyone, and frankly, I've tried to talk to him about his rather careless attitude toward drinking and living. That said, he also, on several occasions, insisted I not discuss any concerns with you, as he intimated you guys were headed in different directions. I did not know you well at all. In fact, I rarely saw you at any events that might have been appropriate for you to join him and where we could get to know each other. I guess for that reason I felt that betraying his confidences and my concerns to someone who in essence was a stranger was not what I should do. I admit that may have been misplaced loyalty, but I believe his current commitment to sobriety and healthier choices will give you both a new starting place in your relationship. How you do it and where it goes is none of my business. I wish you both to be happy in life, as I believe that's all any of us really want. We simply need to get on our own path to that end. I'm sorry I didn't do as well by you as I could have. Thanks for the clothes; I'll get them to him."

I turned and walked down the walk. The afternoon heat and the uncomfortable feeling that I had failed my friend by somehow failing his wife made for as depressing a walk as I had taken in a long time. The heaviness of the humidity did not come close to the heaviness of my soul. I was angry with myself and with Tommy. The damage that fermented liquids reap upon relationships and lives not lived honestly is impossible to overstate. I felt as if I were somehow to blame for my friend's broken self, despite knowing better. "Hell, I'm a doctor; I should be able to fix this" was the unrealistic mantra I had repeated to myself on many an occasion. This was as untrue as Tommy's drunken thinking convincing him that the alcohol gave him a shelter from some pain. Even I knew he needed to confront the pain to find the shelter.

TWENTY-SIX

I RETURNED HOME and got packed. The beauty of this trip was that I had no need for a suit. I had no intention of doing anything more formal than meeting, in casual clothes, with Tommy's therapist or counselor. I wasn't sure of the individual's title, and it didn't really matter if he or she was on team Tommy. I found a couple Columbia fishing shirts and some lightweight cargo pants, threw in a couple of polo shirts and a pair of slacks; a pair of loafers (no socks required); some underwear; and my travel kit containing deodorant, shaving cream, and a hairbrush, and I was packed. I set aside my favorite all-purpose Under Armour tennis shoes to wear on the plane. I then thought of the Ely fishing pamphlet I had found in Kirk's office and retrieved it from my car. This I tossed into my bag with my laptop computer, spare phone charger, and computer charger. I didn't think I would need anything else, and if something came up, I would purchase it there. It wasn't as if I were leaving civilization.

A couple hours later, we were having a family dinner, which I thoroughly enjoyed. This was when I could hear the unfiltered musings from my children without them being relayed to me by Kay later—that being a common occurrence on typical workdays. The major story of the evening was that my daughter felt that the other girls at school were mean for not including a new student in their usual lunch and social group. The girl apparently had an accent, and this was the stain eliciting ostracism by the others. I tried to determine the origin of the accent from my daughter's rendition, but this only led us to laughter. I, having a moment of parental wisdom, pointed out that us laughing at my daughter's attempted accent was as mean as her friends' mocking of the real accent. I then encouraged both kids to embrace the differences in all of us. The world was figuratively getting smaller, and when I traveled to other countries, I was the one with the funny accent and did not want to be made fun of. I wanted them to always be the welcoming ones that made strangers feel like friends. I avoided the lecture on the world also containing bad people and caution being important as well. It is the balancing of these mindsets that distinguishes the true confident individual. I figured I had another year of family meals before tackling the world-as-a-dangerous-place conversation. I sat there smiling and proud of my daughter for her innate goodness—surely an attribute given by her mother.

I got a text from Mike as we were concluding dinner that said he would call when he landed, but it would probably be midafternoon, as he was completing a couple things at work. I looked forward to seeing my buddy. He always made life exciting.

TWENTY-SEVEN

THE FLIGHT WAS uneventful, which is always the goal of anyone boarding a fabricated transportation device—either self-driving car, high-speed rail, or the aluminum sausage with wings that was constructed with some components and labor being contracted out to the lowest bidder. Aviation history overall was very good, but the recent defects of an aircraft allowing a door to take an early exit at sixteen thousand feet over Portland, Oregon, once again pointed out that even with Six Sigma statistical quality, the opportunity for disaster was never going to be zero. That miniscule opportunity to join the pantheon of those that have gone down in such disasters did not ever create any qualms within me. I liked flying. It was the hoards trying to get into or out of the terminals that gave it such a bad name—especially those unaccustomed to the subtle nuances of travel, such as, if you need to hire additional porters for your fifteen pieces of luggage, you haven't thought this out; if your oversize bag comes in at forty-five pounds overweight and you are repacking at the counter, you have not thought this out; and if you are arguing with the employees at the check-in desk that your flight is boarding, and you don't have your ticket, you have not thought this out. Yeah, I love flying, even after witnessing such behavior. *I'm gaining further lessons in patience; I should embrace it*, I thought, heading down the jetway with my bag and laptop case from overhead, easily moving toward my rental car.

The car reserved for me was a KIA Telluride that was a somewhat odd shade of green. The vehicle had a navigation option that I was grateful to have, as I wasn't always sure of cell service in many places I seemed to frequent in my travels. I entered the address for Capital Medical Supply and was directed to head north on 5, then catch Highway 62 to Interstate 35W. The drive was only about thirty minutes, depending on traffic. I was in no hurry. The summertime temperatures in Minnesota were a very pleasant change from those of Florida. The real treat, however, was a level of humidity that wasn't condensing into rivulets on my neck. No, these were the environmental gifts given to those who took the winters in the face without complaint. In fact, they mocked the Gods of the tundra by inventing snowshoes, cross-country skis, and snowmobiles, putting up to three thousand miles a season on such devices. They created heated huts to set upon the ice, allowing them to harvest the lakes' bounty in short sleeves with beer in hand and nary a shiver to the outside temperature of negative twenty degrees Fahrenheit. Yeah, the people of the northern climes deserved and relished their glorious summer respite. I certainly did.

I reached the address without any issues, again thankful for the navigational advantage modern electronics have provided. I slowly drove around the complex. The office was clearly labeled with large signage across the face of three separate office entrances, and to the rear of the park there appeared to be storage spaces that would admit large trucks to pull in and then through. There were three rows of storage places in total, as well as three rows of office condos. I noted one being a logistical company, another a transportation trucking firm, and a smattering of others. The large complex was set off by some significant landscaping in the medians fronting the office condos. There were mature trees along the perimeters, and some cameras were mounted on poles scattered around the perimeter and at the corners of the structures. The office condos all appeared to be one story toward the front, with a second level beginning halfway back on the roof. In those second floors were some small windows. I didn't see any external doors or fire escapes, but I suspected the need of fire exits and surmised that the doors may have been hidden by architectural design.

It was early afternoon, and I had grabbed a sandwich in the concourse before getting to the car rental agency, so I selected a spot in the shade of a tree and thought I would see just how busy the home office of Capital Medical was. I was considering the attributes of my turkey and provolone sandwich when I saw a Jeep pull to the front of the office. I nearly spit out my half-chewed bite when I realized the figure exiting the Jeep was Kirk, our MIA perfusionist. He glanced around briefly, then entered the center door of the three labeled with the Capital Medical signage. I had no time to consider this and its implications, as my phone erupted in its musical awakening. I looked at the screen and saw Mike's profile image appear. I spoke into the phone as my sense of stability was trying to correct this reality distortion, even though I was firmly ensconced in my rental car with a partially consumed sandwich, both now seemingly desultory activities frozen in time.

"Mike, are you close by? You aren't going to believe what I think I just saw," I spoke into the atmosphere of the car's interior.

"Well, I'm leaving the airport and going to make a couple stops on the way. I have some people I want to talk to and need to pick up a couple of things. I have the hotel you are staying at in Center City and made a reservation for tonight. Can I meet you there, say, around seven?"

I quickly replied, "Sure, no problem. We can grab dinner, and I can pick your brain on this circus."

He then realized I had said he wouldn't believe what I had seen. "Ben, what is it you saw or are seeing?"

"Mike, it was our chief perfusionist, Kirk, walking into the distributor of our heparin—the drug I believe is causing the issues," I answered.

"Well, if he is the chief, he may have been looking into this as well, though it seems like a leap to have an employee dog-paddling in the water where the feds are swimming. I think I may have some information that could help you, but we can talk about it tonight. You aren't planning on going into those offices too, I hope?" he asked.

"I haven't decided yet, but I think I will try to talk to Kirk when he comes out," I said softly, though no one was in earshot other than Mike. I recognized my nerves were a touch on edge. I had not yet put the presence of Kirk in the grab bag of things I had expected to see on my stakeout. I guess the movies had this scenario all the time. You would think I would have been prepared. Life imitating art, as it were. Mike and I ended our conversation with his admonition not to go into the office and to note if surveillance cameras were watching me watch. I considered that good advice from a spy, so I looked carefully, 360 degrees around my KIA. I didn't think I had missed any on my parking lot cruise.

Kirk exited the building about fifteen minutes later and got into his Jeep. I pulled out of my space and trailed after him as he went through the exit to the frontage road off the interstate. After a couple blocks, I sped up, pulled in front of him, and stopped quickly.

I realized I had cut him close; he very easily could have rear-ended me and added to my list of issues. I started to get out, but Kirk was already out of his vehicle with a 9mm Sig Sauer in his hand. I exited the KIA. "Jesus, Kirk; it's me, Ben. What are you doing here, and what's with the gun?" I quickly asked. I recognized the gun as his from our shared time at the range. It was a good carry weapon a little smaller than my Glock but weighing about the same, at twenty-two to twenty-three ounces with the magazine in. He had a seventeen-round magazine in his, and I had no doubt it was loaded.

"Ben, what the hell are you doing here?" He continued to hold the gun, though now pointed downward and next to his thigh to avoid any passing car onlooker anxiety. I felt that the answering ball was in my court. "I'm up here to see Tommy but thought I'd visit the heparin distributor and see if I can figure out where the presumably contaminated heparin came from and how we fit into this. It seems more complicated than just a bad batch of a common drug. Let's go grab a coffee, and you can tell me what you are doing in their office and anything else that might help solve this mystery."

"I'll google a Starbucks. Just a minute," he said, replacing his Sig in a belly band holster beneath his generous untucked shirt. Knowing the gun was there, I still would have been hard pressed to call him out on it being evident.

A couple of minutes later, we had decided on a Starbucks about a mile from the industrial park and adjacent to the University of Minnesota campus. Fifteen minutes later, we were sitting outside at a shaded table with our coffees. It appeared that most of the locals wanted the sun-exposed seats. This the inverse of the general order of things in Florida, where shade is the desired site of respite.

TWENTY-EIGHT

EMMA SAT IN the depressing log room in an even more depressed mood. The darkened veil across her limited vision was being lifted gently by the first streaking rays of gold. The earlier application of mosquito repellent was now only a minor impedance to the buzzing swarm that was rallying around her. The swatting and scratching were now reaching the threshold of maddening hysteria. She was unsure whether she wanted to eat or simply surrender herself to the likelihood of death by either insect or human torture. At some point, it might not matter. She wasn't stupid. She recognized the brain trust of the pervert eyebrow guy and Marathon Man were incapable of planning whatever this was, and she was still uncertain why they felt she should be a part of it. She wondered briefly whether offering herself sexually would provide an escape option, however unlikely. She suspected eyebrows paid for his sexual encounters with a Toys "R" Us credit card.

She had inherited seven hundred thousand dollars from the death of her mother several years earlier, and when the perfusion job in the beach town opened, she got hired and moved. Her inheritance had allowed her to purchase the condo from an estate that simply was trying to divest assets for the far-flung heirs. They accepted her lowball offer, and there she was. She worked to pay the real-estate taxes, which were reasonable, as she had homesteaded the property, thus minimizing the annual escalation seen across Florida. The HOA fees, however, were not capped, and it seemed as if the cost of maintaining the lawns, community pool, clubhouse, and roofs of the units was untethered to real dollars and more akin to Monopoly money. She was convinced the presence of a hurricane somewhere in the world had a direct impact on her association dues. She understood the risk of the insurance companies, but the system was now a disaster before the state had a disaster. These ridiculous sidebar thoughts were frequently hijacking her attempts to understand her current circumstance. Maybe the mosquito torture was inducing some cerebral dysfunction. *Focus, damn it! Skip the why and think about the what next. You must get yourself out of it!* She brought herself back to the present and convinced herself to try and be more pleasant to her captor when he brought the next meal and took her to the outhouse. He had been minimally responsive thus far, but she felt at some level he was a much better option than Marathon Man. She would look for some stick or stone that might offer utilization as a weapon. It wouldn't be much against the gun, but if she got in the first blow, who knew. If nothing else, it was a distraction to think about this option as opposed to the constant scratching. She needed more repellent and would beg for it if need be.

A short time later, the sun was fully washing the landscape with a warm morning glow as she heard the footfalls of the perv. The direction to "get away from the door" followed closely. She readily complied, and the door slowly opened. She noted for the first time that he brought his gun hand though the threshold first before the door was fully opened. She replayed the earlier entrances and was convinced this was his "style"—and not a good one. She realized it might offer an opportunity for a confrontation she could utilize.

She had taken some self-defense classes in college a few years ago and recalled the instructor saying that if the attacker was reacting to pain, his focus was lost, at least momentarily. It would be during the follow-up moment that she would have to improvise. Perhaps it was a glimmer of hope and not much more, but it was something. She would rehearse her moves between meals.

She walked the path toward the outhouse and frankly thought she would much rather complete her business in the woods to avoid the omnipresent flies and mosquitos in the rancid structure. She imagined the locals utilizing such conveniences selectively, retreating to the woods until a good freeze cleared the unwanted airborne observers of bodily functions. She continuously scanned the ground for something that might become a weapon upon her escape. She noted a reasonably stout stick lying next to the path almost to the outhouse. It was to her right, which would allow her to grasp it and swing quickly if possible. She entered the box of white-noise buzzing and quickly completed her task and used the sandpaper-quality paper to wipe. This brought itching and irritation to the one place that had avoided the biting tormentors. This was really a cruel joke, and she felt as if God were somehow taunting her. Then she retracted the thought as she realized she would be calling on God soon if she were to try and escape.

She tried to move her ass a little as she looked over her shoulder to the perv and tried to beg as enticingly as possible for the chance to get more repellent applied. The caterpillar brows seemed focused on her ass, so while doing this, she showed her swollen, blotchy forearm, which negated any sexual inuendo. There were some obstacles to every plan, but you have to play the cards you have. To her relief, the perv called out and the cabin door opened, with a new persona standing in the shadow of the porch. This guy also displayed the facial features of Asian descent and was maybe five feet seven inches in height. Emma thought she had a solid two to three inches on him. That somehow made her feel a sense of superiority that, while strictly imaginary, was a good feeling, nonetheless. He, too, sported a short haircut, but with a wannabe mullet that seemed to shorten his stature by its presence. Maybe it did so by making his thick neck look shorter, thus providing little room between his head and shoulders. She wondered if he was missing some cervical vertebrae. His arms were exposed, and as he tossed the repellent to Emma, she saw that he sported a red dragon tattoo on his right forearm. As she was applying it, Mullet Man stepped into the cabin and retrieved a tray of food, which included an egg. She hoped to hell it was hard boiled, as the shell was on it, and she could imagine the "joke" of cracking the shell to find it not cooked. The tray also held a bottle of water and a piece of bread. A Michelin four-star meal to be sure. She held the tray disguised as a plastic plate and returned down the path. Mullet Man had not uttered a word. She wondered where Marathon Man was and whether there were more of these jerks around. It appeared she was attending the local Asian social club outing.

TWENTY-NINE

THE COFFEES WERE only partially consumed as Kirk began. "Ben, I think I may have been the source of the bad heparin. When I went to China, I met a guy named Jin Lee. He was our 'guide' provided by the communist government to ensure we didn't somehow get crossways with local authorities. He was cool and didn't seem to be caught up in the whole political program, if you know what I mean. If he heard one of us getting into some political conversation or even expressing a negative opinion of the treatment of the Uyghurs or suppression of Tibetan culture, he would put his fingers to his lips, say shush, and walk away. He knew we would continue the conversation, but he did not want to be implicated in any way with such revolutionary thoughts that could easily result in harsh reprisals from the party. We got along well and talked about fishing and the places we had been He told me he had been fishing here in Minnesota a couple of times and told me of outfitters and guides north of here he had used. We subsequently met and had a four-day trip into the Boundary Waters Canoe Area Wilderness here in Minnesota. He arranged the trip from China, including a guide, equipment, and the required permits. I was impressed by his logistical prowess. It would have taken some effort from me, living in the States and only one time zone different. Anyway, while I was in China and then on the fishing trip, we talked about how cardiac cases were done here in the States and the problems we were having in keeping a reliable source of medicines, particularly heparin. On the China trip, he said he worked with the provider of the heparin that we used. He thought the company could easily ship to the US if they weren't already. I said we would be interested if it was okay with Howard in Pharmacy, as he would understand the regulations et cetera. Howard said we were already using heparin manufactured in China, as that was the primary source of the world's supply. I contacted Jin. He got us set up with a delivery schedule through the distributor here, Capital Medical. We put the orders into them, and the drugs came as promised. Jin got us a discounted price, and Howard and I split the savings we paid versus the old, invoiced price. It wasn't a great deal of money; I think I made twenty-five to thirty thousand last year from the deal. That didn't get me rich, but it helped the cause. I let Howard handle the invoices, and I never saw what he had them marked as for accounting. It may have been more, but I didn't want to know. I felt like I was in deep enough, and I guess I thought ignorance was somehow defensible."

"Well, that explains your presence here. Did you learn anything from Capital Medical? Was Emma involved in this? Did Howard do any other drug deals with this guy Jin? How long has this been going on?" I spewed forth all these questions before Kirk could reply. "Okay, I'm sorry for the verbal diarrhea. First off, was Emma involved in this?" I inquired, with calm restored to my thinking. I realized I had sounded like a first-year medical student seeing a C-section and asking how that baby got there—a totally absurd lack of precision thinking.

"I told Emma of the small side deal, and since she frequently retrieved the drugs and interacted with Howard, I thought she should be included. For the last few months, we would split my portion of the money we received in the difference between the invoiced price and the actual payment. This money was sent to an account from Jin through a bank here in Minnesota, always in amounts less than five thousand, avoiding any IRS scrutiny and not appearing as a flag to the bank. Emma seemed okay with it, and she had never personally met Jin. I didn't think this would turn out to be such a cluster. I haven't been able to reach Emma, and I don't know if she took off scared or there is something else going on. I heard she was in the car with Tommy ... Sorry, Dr. Moore."

"He's Tommy to his friends, and I'm sure that includes you. I don't think Emma going missing is related to Tommy and the infamous car ride. I am afraid it is somehow tied up in this drug hustle you have going. That said, I'm unclear as to what her running or being taken gets her or whoever kidnapped her. I do believe she is still alive if it is related to the drug deal and not some whack job psycho that fell in love with her in the produce section of the grocery store and felt she should be with him for eternity. So back to Howard. Do you think he could have expanded the drug options available for price skimming?"

Kirk paused and then offered, "I wouldn't be surprised. I got the sense he needed as opposed to wanted the money. One day when I was picking up some drugs from the stock room, he came in and asked if I thought Jin would be available to talk to him. I thought it odd because Howard had spoken to him by phone when this got started and I kind of had the impression they had met in person at some point. I know Howard made a trip to China with his wife a couple years ago, so I thought they may have been part of the same sort of group I was with on the medical mission,

Howard being there to evaluate pharmacies. I never really talked to him about it, as I didn't want to say anything that would lead him to think I organized this."

"How did Jin get you to consider this?" I asked, looking him directly in the eyes, wondering if there might be something yet unsaid.

"When we were fishing up here in Minnesota, we got to talking about the shortage of drugs worldwide and the difficulty we were having in securing a consistent source of heparin. He said his contacts in China could provide us with heparin and other drugs we might need. He said that if I wanted, he could help us set up an account with Capital Medical distributors here in the twin cities. They would manage our orders and ensure delivery. He then mentioned the improved price to us as a favored friend and now customer. He explained how, by buying through his group of manufacturers, shipping, and a stateside distributor, we would be saving money, and in fact he suggested I have my own little company that could take advantage of the price difference, and we all would make money on the deal. When I got back to Florida, I met with Howard and laid out the option of getting some of our inventory from Jin through Capital Medical. He asked about the pricing and then said that if we got it cheaper, we should keep the difference for our efforts in helping the hospital system. I was frankly shocked by his willingness to do this. I didn't know him that well but thought this to be out of character. The coincidence that both he and Jin suggested we skim the deal seemed like a sign that I should do it. In retrospect, I have a feeling, as I said, that they knew each other and I was the mark, so to speak. That may sound self-serving, and, I know, at a minimum unethical, if not illegal, but here we are."

"Did your trip to China occur before or after Howard's?" I asked.

"It was shortly after, I believe" was his reply.

"How did you and Jin decide to meet to fish here in Minnesota? It seems awfully fortuitous that you are meeting relatively close to his stateside distributor. Though I guess they could have suggested the fishing site to him as a perk to one of their customers."

"I got a text message from Jin a month or so after I got back from the China trip. He asked if I would like to meet up here for a few days of walleye fishing. I said it sounded great. He offered to arrange guides and lodging. This was about two years ago. We arranged to meet in Ely, about four hours northwest of here. This was when the deal came together from his standpoint, and when I returned, Howard was on board, as I said."

"Where did you stay in Ely?" I asked, though not sure it mattered.

"Jin had rented an incredibly beautiful cabin on one of the boundary waters entrance lakes, Fall Lake. He was there with a couple of people he introduced as executives of the heparin manufacturing facility and one from Capital Medical. The guide met us there on the first trip. We headed north up the lake, and after a short portage you are in the Boundary Waters Canoe Area Wilderness. We fished three days and stayed in a couple different campsites. Then we came back out again into Fall Lake. The Capital Medical guy—John was his name—stayed with one of the heparin executives another day, as they said their permit was independent of ours and they held a longer stay option. I never saw John or the heparin guy again on that trip or the next. When I asked today at Capital Medical to speak to John, they said there was no one by that name on the payroll. So, I thought I would leave and try to figure this out. You were in the parking lot, and I still haven't gotten any of this solved about the bad heparin or who the hell I fished with by the name of John." He sounded quite frustrated. There was an anger and unease smoldering beneath Kirk's portrayed emotions, and I felt he was coming to understand there was potentially something sinister in the activities of his business associate Jin and maybe Howard.

I shared his concerns but nonetheless tried to reassure him of the probability something benign was the answer. Addressing him, I said, "I think you should get back to Florida and try to inventory the heparin we got sent. See if Howard cooperates in the effort. I know the FDA wants to speak to all who handled the product, and your absence seems to raise red flags that we don't want to deal with. I have a meeting tomorrow with Tommy and his therapist to help him deal with whatever issues I might have some knowledge of, given the many years of our friendship. I was going to ask about our heparin shipments at Capital Medical, but given what you told me, I think I'll hold off on that. What do you think, Kirk? Sound like a plan?"

"Yeah, it makes the most sense. I want to see the records Howard kept of our orders. I know the pharmacy is busy, but it seemed as if the delivery dock was much more active the last few months. I don't know what I think, but something there is bothering me. I suppose being here doesn't help or answer those questions. I'll see about trying to get back tonight or on an early a.m. flight."

"I think that's the best idea. Kirk, if you need to talk to a lawyer, Tommy's guy, Wyatt Slife, is terrific. And if you say I sent you, I believe he'll take extra care of you." We sat silent for a moment as we both contemplated the near unknown future. I broke the silence with "This will get straightened out. I believe you were at least partially victimized here, and it pisses me off that somehow our patients are paying the price for the shortcomings of the system. The commitment is to provide the caregivers with the tools required to save lives—not just a few lives, but thousands daily. We will get to the bottom of this, I promise." I left unsaid the dark foreboding I harbored over the situation with Emma.

We parted shortly after this, as Kirk found a flight to Florida on his Delta app that was leaving in a couple hours. I decided I would head up to Center City. My reservations were at an Inn in St Croix Falls, Wisconsin, about ten miles east of Center City. I was on Highway 8, nearing Center City, when my phone interrupted my contemplation of the upcoming meeting with Tommy's therapist and, more importantly, of my helplessness in finding out anything regarding Emma's disappearance.

THIRTY

MY PHONE DISPLAYED Mike's face as I answered. "Ben where are you?" was his perfunctory greeting.

"I'm twenty to thirty minutes from the inn. How about you? Are you close?" I responded.

"I'm just getting out of the cities, so I would guess I'm an hour out. Let's meet at the inn—I have some information we should discuss—and then grab dinner."

"Sounds good. Anything we can talk about now, or should it wait?" I asked.

His quick response of "It should wait" carried the hint of quiet concern over the news he was bringing.

"Sounds like a plan. I'll see you in about an hour," I confirmed, and we disconnected. I drove a few miles and then called Kirk, who was nearing the airport. "Kirk, you mentioned the cabin you stayed at on Fall Lake. Did you stay there both times?" I asked.

"Yes, we did. The second trip after we got back from the Boundary Waters, we took some of the fish to the guide's cabin on a smaller lake near Fall Lake. I believe it was called Cedar Lake. There was no road to his cabin. He kept a small runabout with a twenty-five-horse Evinrude on his trailer. We helped him get it into the water at a small ramp where he then parked his truck in the trees, mostly out of sight, and took us and the fish to his cabin on the other side of the lake and down what seemed like a couple of miles from the ramp. The cabin was rustic and would have been harsh in winter but still a great setup if you didn't like neighbors or noise other than the wildlife. He told us he stayed there most of the year but took a couple months off in winter to fish the gulf from Florida to Texas—depending on his mood, I guess. That whole ecosystem is pretty much the redneck riviera. If you like fried food, slow talk, beer, and the southern perspective of life and the government's ruining of it, it's okay. I've fished there a few times but never really felt like the locals cared one way or another if you were there with some money to spend or not. They simply tolerated you." This was more information than I had asked for, but having some sense of who Kirk had met and what they were like seemed like good intel to collect.

"Was the guide an okay dude? Do you think he and Jin were somehow connected beyond client and guide?" I asked.

Kirk replied, "I think the guide was okay. He seemed like a normal Midwestern outdoorsman. I also sensed he wasn't particularly fond of the Chinese. We talked around the campfires and in the boat while fishing. He would push Jin on 'made in China' labels as being a warning, only half joking. He also surprised me in wanting to have Jin explain Chinese foreign policy based on the 'Belt and Road Initiative.' The guide seemed disturbed that the Chinese government was simply loaning susceptible countries large sums of money that their leaders either embezzled, wasted, or spent on projects with little or no oversight that were completed by Chinese laborers. The countries then owed the Chinese incredible debts. These debts then called by way of land for outposts, naval ports, or mineral rights. He seemed truly incensed by these policies, and I was surprised. It seemed out of character for the quintessential fishing guide. I guess internet access, even in northern Minnesota, provided the opportunity for expansion of worldviews. Jin tried to defend his country's largesse but didn't seem all that married to the party line. His questions always revolved around the Boundary Waters north and south of the US Canadian border. He was curious as to how it was patrolled, how the permits were granted, and where and how long the portages were. Occasionally he would ask about fishing the waters, but the geography and ecology seemed more interesting to him, as I recall. In retrospect, it was a lot of intellectual conversation and atmosphere on those trips."

"Do you have a contact for your guide?" I asked.

"I do or did. I have tried a few times over the last year to get him on the phone with no luck. I've left messages and expected a call back but never got it. The last couple times, it said the number was not in service. Not sure what happened to him."

"Do you have a last name or outfitter that he worked through?"

"I believe his last name was Harty or Haywood—something like that," came the reply. "I'm close to the airport in some traffic. If I think of anything else about the guy, I'll give you a call." And the conversation ended.

I pulled into St. Croix Falls, WI. It had the charm of an old river town with the sheen of a well marketed new generation. The storefronts were updated, and the enticement of outdoor activities around the river and valley were hard to ignore. It looked like a great small, family-oriented town from the outside. I wondered whether the scourge of drugs had contaminated the idyllic facade I had so quickly assigned this place. I hoped not. I wanted to believe there were, yet some bastions of unvarnished values tainted only by awareness and not consumption. They resisted the overwhelming tsunami consuming all of America—the seemingly universal desire to feel no pain, face no adversity, and live without demands or consequences put upon us. We had become a utopia-seeking society, and that quest was destroying large numbers of us daily. We demanded no physical pain following surgery or the consequences of accidents of our own making or that of others. We bought into the swan song of the pharma sales reps, those Harold Hill–like pied piper peddlers that prowled the corridors of hospitals and doctor' offices across the country. Their seventy-six-trombone medley was that pain was easily obliterated by pills with no consequences, much in the same way that the instrument-playing townsfolk of Meredith Wilson's *The Music Man* required no practice. The late realization of the medical community and of society as to this fallacy was as distorting and damaging as the equivalent of a hundred 9/11s every year.

I shook myself free of this maudlin train of thought and exited the car, immediately noting the summer Midwestern humidity. While no match for that of Florida, it was still a reminder that deodorant was recommended for the benefit of others. I exited the rental and observed the western horizon lifting dark gray pillars of clouds topped with rolling pregnant blue-green caps that seemed to spill over those shifting pillars and extend the growing column to yet higher reaches as I watched. The delivery of this atmospheric fetus would be a relief to the water-starved farmers yet anxiety provoking because of the potential damage of wind and hail. This was going to be a storm as intense as one could imagine. While generally short in duration, these summer maelstroms with their chaotic freight-train-force winds, when focused on a structure, can render it a scattered heap of its component parts miles from its origin. I had these similar thoughts as a youth growing up in an

Iowa farming community. That dependence of the farmers, their families, and communities for their livelihood on the benevolence of the weather solidified my desire to pursue another vocation. I was glad not to be venturing out on the roads or water in the path of this impending event. I checked into my room, which was a small standalone cabin. It was clean and rustic with faux logs on the front. A microwave sat on a counter, with a coffee maker adjacent. They offered free internet access and a TV with limited cable channels. Some options included RFD-TV, HGTV, and The History Channel, next to CNN, Fox News, and ESPN—all demographics satisfied.

I called Kay. I wanted to hear about her day and the kids. That was the tonic of choice for me. But I was also looking forward to a scotch with dinner and a catch-up conversation with Mike. This seemed a bit duplicitous in that I was going to be visiting my partner in the morning in his quest to kick his addiction to alcohol. The nearness of the disease of alcoholism caused me some introspection on my own use and occasional abuse of the substance. It is a fine line that seems to separate the acknowledged afflicted from the rest.

THIRTY-ONE

FORTY-FIVE MINUTES LATER, Mike called. I was looking at a map of Minnesota I had gotten in the office as I checked in. It displayed the boundary area with Canada. I was trying to get a sense of the fishing location Kirk had described. Answering the phone, I appreciated the wool-like grayness cloaking my cabin through the window. Simultaneously I heard a dull, reverberating roll of thunder. The storm would soon be delivering its payload of moisture and wind to the citizens and visitors with me in this little valley of the river. Being on the Badger side or the Gopher side of this mascot-dividing waterway would be of no consequence or hindrance to this storm, as had been so for any storm that had crossed the great prairies for millennia. This arbitrary delineation of property tax recipients held no meaning to nature. It was as meaningless as the treaties with the Native Americans were—those tribes who preceded the surveyors' tripod-mounted theodolite. Nature, and historically the earliest settlers, didn't care about ownership of land. They cared only about what was beneath the falling rain, blowing wind, or shuffling feet of the farmer trying to break the surface crust into accepting the seeds of a potential crop. The rain started to strike the roof and widows, The temperature immediately cooled, and the stiletto shards of lightning streaked the sky, accompanied by their dance partners, the wall-shaking, resonating booms of thunder. The sound and feel of the air compression as direct as the amplified chords of AC/DC playing "Thunderstruck."

"Mike," I answered, "Are you responsible for bringing this storm with you?"

His chuckled reply was "No, but I think you might be involved in another kind of storm as well. That one may have an impact that should give you pause."

"I'm intrigued. Are you here at the inn?" I asked.

"Yeah, got in about ten minutes ago. Just beat the rain as I came east on Highway 8."

"Let's meet in the office in an hour to give this storm time to move through. The clerk can give us a dinner recommendation," I offered.

"Sounds like a plan. I guess if the warning sirens go off, best to head into the bathroom, huh," he stated somewhat hesitantly. He followed with "I don't see any storm shelters in my room. How about yours?"

"None in mine either. It's either the bathroom or the closet I guess," I replied. "Let's hope the only reason to go to the bathroom is to relieve ourselves before dinner."

"Agreed," he concluded. "See you in an hour."

Being an expert on short naps as required to get through residency, and possessing the blessed ability to ignore any distractions, I promptly laid down on the bed, confident today's storm did not intend to collect me for the march to the afterlife. The storm Mike had mentioned for some reason seemed far more threatening. That, however, would wait until after my nap. My phone alarm set, I was asleep inside of three minutes. This was a gift many people envied—particularly if they were in the same room and had to listen to my snoring. Those unfortunate souls prayed for the two-minute magic to come to them.

The alarm brought me abruptly awake and focused—again the residual effect of many nights of patient demands. I suspected I would maintain this trait long after I retired. I brushed my teeth and hair, and cracked the door to see it was no longer raining and the air remained cool. A partial rainbow hung in the west, refracting the slanted rays of the horizon-bound sun. The storm had collected the humidity in its marauding assault eastward and left a residual environment reminiscent of coastal California. There was a gentle breeze, the plants and grass glistening under the translucent coating of the rain, and the subtle call of the distant blackbirds near the river, with the closer low but distinct mourning dove cooing. The unique whistling sound of their wings as they took off and landed in the wires and trees near the inn gave the impression and reminder that most life continued undisturbed by the passing weather. There appeared to have been no local wind damage, thus—at least on the Badger side of the river—life was moving on, grateful for the rain without the accompanying destruction that had circulated nearby.

I stepped into the office. Mike was there, and we exchanged the expected but genuine "bro" hug. Mike was just getting the clerk's recommendation for dinner, which would include a good piece of Midwestern corn-fed beef and a drink. The clerk seemed to have no hesitancy in the direction he was sending us. Mike slipped him a couple bucks for the information, and we headed for the door. It had been ten or eleven months since M.D. and I had seen each other. I looked him over as we approached his rental four-wheel-drive SUV. His hair was a little long, with its ever-present curl. I always wondered if this was supported by some magical product that we mere mortals, facing the typical aging of our cranial fur piece (i.e., thinning, and stiffening while transforming to a greying cover) could only envy. I tried to look closely and thought he might have a couple strands of the gray stuff there, but it was not detracting from the semiwild shock adorning his smiling countenance. He appeared not to have gained any weight or lost any of his musculature in the interval since our last reunion. No, M.D. seemed to be that individual that time and its erosive effects would largely ignore until the final days.

As we neared the vehicle, dodging the variously sized puddles in the pockmarked parking lot, he asked how I did at the range. "I don't seem to have lost anything with the Glock, and in fact I feel like in the last year I've improved my distance accuracy quite a bit. What about you? Are you still imagining the day you outshoot me?" I chided, this last being a hollow statement of my persistent place of second in our shooting competitions.

"Just curious. I grabbed a couple of weapons from our local office and thought we either might need them or can see if you are still that marine character you play on TV," he laughingly responded.

"While I appreciate your recognition of my unblemished and stellar marine service, your comment about 'might need' the weapons leads me to believe we need to talk," I answered, immediately feeling akin to most wives wanting some face time with a spouse or partner who is ignoring their primal concerns, whatever they might be at that moment.

"Ben, you are spot on. We do need to talk over a steak and a beer," he replied as we entered the SUV and Mike chauffeured us to the recommended haunt to satisfy our hunger.

THIRTY-TWO

EMMA SAT ON the bed, awaiting the arrival of Mr. Perv, and tried to imagine the opportunity to set about an escape. The afternoon had brought a short but relatively fierce thunderstorm. The air in the cabin seemed fresher and cooler by several degrees. While this was welcome, it in no way negated the odor she was sure was emanating from the folds of her body. Since the hand pump in the cabin was not working, there was no rinsing of bra or any other piece of nearly week-worn clothing. She thought that while the perv might lust after her from afar, any close encounters would surely shrivel his manhood via aromatic poison. The combination of dried blood, perspiration, and mosquito repellant had to be listed on the governmental toxic dump lists and entitle her to federal cleanup funds. The thought of this gave her some temporary mental delight as she envisioned such a list of rank individuals. While it might be a reasonable defensive strategy to ward off rape, she understood that the male driven to sexual assault was not likely to be deterred by a cloak of eye-watering odor coming from a female form. The old joke about sheep fuckers, if true, would seem to confirm this fact. She went back to contemplating an escape scenario, but given the established routine, she was depressed by what little chance she had before her. She decided that she would see if they would let her walk down to the lake to at least splash some water. A short time later, the shuffling footfalls of her jailor, the Perv, were heard on the trail coming toward her. It was a little early for dinner but probably within the realm of possibility.

The command to step back was barked again with the lilt of a Scandinavian accent which was so incongruous to the Asiatic features that produced it that she knew without seeing him utter the words. The door lock rattled, and then the door cracked. Again, she noted that the gun preceded any other body part, including breast-fixated eyes, of this human connection to the world beyond these confining walls. There was no tray of food, only the motioned arm swing with the gun directing her to start up the trail. "While we are having this stroll, would you please take me to the lake to rinse off a little? I know I smell like a compost pile in the barnyard, so we would both benefit from just a little attention to some hygiene. That okay with you?" she stated, trying to sound friendly.

His reply of "We'll see" was as noncommittal as a press release from the White House responding to the question of who the president's favorite senator was. They arrived at the main cabin, and the door opened to allow Marathon Man and Mullet Man to come onto the porch and sit in front of her, while the Perv remained behind her. Mullet Man quietly asked her what had happened to their drugs. Her immediate thought and response were of confusion.

"I'm not sure. We are still using the heparin we are getting, and I presume it is from you guys. So, I think the drugs are where they are supposed to be—in the Pharmacy storage space."

The two men before her looked a little baffled initially, and then an angry eruption from marathon man. "We don't give a shit aboot your heparin. What happened to the fentanyl?"

The dynamics of her circumstances came immediately into focus for Emma. The heparin hustle was somehow related but inconsequential to the goonies before her and their very lucrative and risky business of major drug smuggling. Why they thought she was involved in that was as absurd as it was frightening. "Listen, guys, I think you have made a mistake here. I don't know anything about fentanyl or any other drugs beyond what we use for our pump patients. Why do you think I would know about this?" she asked, again trying to remain composed in the face of what was now a very delicate situation. She wanted to scream at these idiots. They kidnapped someone with no knowledge of their business. Somebody, to the best of her recollection, got stabbed for the effort, and they were wasting time sitting with her in some primitive green acre, hoping she would give them the whereabouts of their products. The realization hit her that if she convinced them she had no information about their drugs or business, she would be of no use to them and, in fact, a liability. This clarity came in a crush of pent-up emotions, frustration, and fear. She quickly determined she had to try and give the impression that she had value, if not information, at least for now. "You know, I think your fentanyl may have gotten mislabeled at receiving," she hypothesized. She really had no idea if the drugs were being shipped to the hospital and were even a part of the heparin deal, she and Kirk were running. It then came to her. *Howard.* He must have been using Kirk and her as shields. They would get the heparin and use the inflated invoices to get the profit out of the system. He could easily have mixed in other receivables, such as fentanyl, and gotten them on the dock and taken to storage, where he had control. They could be taken out and handed to whomever, and he was only the middleman. She suspected Howard had either seen what she and Kirk were doing and amplified it, or he somehow arranged for Kirk to meet the Chinese guy, Jin, whom she had never met, and put the whole deal in motion. She was not sure how he felt Kirk's participation would enhance the deal other than to provide cover for the distributor, Capital Medical, here in the States. As she got to this conclusion in seconds, she knew that was the answer. *We had to be getting products from Capital Medical to allow the addition of the narcotics to the shipment. Capital was the central figure in this.*

"As we sit here. I think I might know what happened to your drugs, or at least where they may have been. You have kept me here so long the situation may have changed. Maybe we can help each other. Eh?" As she spoke, she did her new impression of the Scandinavian brough she kept hearing in their voices. She was trying to formulate a plan that would provide her with the chance to escape. She was not a camper, and her knowledge of the wooded hills and valleys was what might be gleaned from a story out of *People* magazine or gathered from a movie like *The Revenant*, where the DiCaprio character is mauled by a bear and left for dead. That was a reality she suspected befell most every lost soul in the North American wilderness, and it was probably worse in Canada, to her way of thinking. They had more bears and fewer people than the US. She hoped she was in the US. As this stream of thought jettisoned through her brain, she heard Mullet Man ask how she could help them. The pregnant pause in her response seemed to extend into another day. "That's a good question. But first tell me how often you speak to Howard."

This out-of-context response seemed to catch the two dark-eyed threats in front of her off balance. "We don't speak to him," Mullet Man replied. "Our associate does. He is the one who is most insistent we get your information, as it seems your friend Howard is unable to communicate with us. We are told the authorities like the FDA are shining lights up your Howard's ass."

Emma was struck by this comment. "You must mean the DEA. They deal in narcotic smuggling. The FDA is in control of prescription drugs." As the words exited her mouth, she knew Kirk and the heparin must have somehow gotten somebody's attention. *Shit, I'm going to die for the crime of impeding a drug smuggler's sales force in the name of a few bucks and blood thinner. The ultimate thinned blood is most likely to be mine, either by the Swedish Chinese or some rando bear in the woods.* "Listen, if it's the FDA, this will get resolved pretty quickly," she lied, knowing the response time of any federal bureaucracy was benchmarked against glacial movement, not the universal minutes, hours, days and so forth. No, the chances of Emma having her seventy-fifth birthday here in the woods was greater than the feds completing an assigned investigation in under three years. "I need to talk to my partner in Florida. Between us we can figure out how to get your drugs out of reach of the FDA." This was another lie, but it was a start.

"We will talk aboot it. Go back to your cabin," Mullet Man commanded.

Emma recognized that this was not the time to press about the lake bath, so that they might, under compassionate prisoner protocol, allow some more mosquito repellent to be used for her benefit and, if nothing else, minimize the offensive odor she knew she was spreading as discreetly as a pheromone-excreting rabbit in heat. The nearly empty spray can was tossed in her direction; she suspected this was as much for their benefit as hers. *The eau de toilette with Deet. The perfect Christmas gift for your girl of the north woods or Everglades. She will always remember you fondly.* She generously sprayed and prayed for relief from all the threatening pests.

THIRTY-THREE

THE RESTAURANT WAS done in a rustic outdoors-themed motif. A large, symmetrical ten-point antler rack hung majestically over a stone fireplace mantel. The main dining room had seven or eight round tables beyond a generously provisioned salad bar. There were a couple of smaller rooms along one side that apparently allowed more discreet dining and conversation. To the other side, a passageway led to the bar, where muffled voices blended with the chords of Toby Keith's' "Should've Been a Cowboy." I was truly appreciating the dining recommendation, and I hadn't yet had anything to eat or drink.

"Okay, big guy, let's talk. What do you know that I should know?" I asked as the waitress took our drink orders. We both selected a single-malt scotch from their slightly limited offerings of the chosen beverage.

The waitress glided away as Mike looked around and then began. "I asked some of my fed colleagues across a couple institutional departments. Interestingly, there was a fair amount of information regarding this neck of the woods and what is believed to be a significant new and increasingly utilized portal for illegal drugs. The reason this is notable is that there is actual communication between the branches of Homeland Security Investigations, who deal in cross-border threats; the DEA; the FBI task force on cartel interdiction and disruption; the border patrol agents locally; state law enforcement agencies; and the northern tier governors who have quietly been sharing information and resources."

"Why haven't I heard or seen any of this in the press?" I asked.

"Look around you. The dealers and distributors are most likely involved in the tourist industry. The hunting, fishing and winter sport economy make a huge impact on the area. The concern about blowback and economic impact has created the agreed need for subtlety. I realize that will only last until some politician can garner face time with an explosive claim of stopping the tons of drugs at the border or excoriating the other party for failing to do it. The current atmosphere of mutual assistance is refreshing and, from what I hear, much appreciated by those on the ground."

"While this is somewhat shocking, I don't think our heparin issue rises to the same impact as the narco traffickers. Do they think the heparin is tied to the more traditional drugs of heroin, fentanyl, oxy, and all the rest?" I asked, a little dumbstruck by what I was learning.

"The story my buddies have developed, and this comes as a consequence of your heparin issue, is that the heparin transaction was a trial balloon, if you will. They wanted to see how difficult it would be to bring things south as opposed to north. They needed to create reliable checkpoints and end points that could avoid scrutiny and yet get them the volume that rewards with big dollars. The information you gave me about Capital Medical was a new avenue for the good guys to pursue. How it plays out, or even if they are involved, remains to be seen."

"I appreciate the information. So how do we go further in trying to get this sorted out? And more importantly, how does the perfusionist, Emma, fit in this, and how do we find her?" I asked, somewhat pleadingly.

Looking at me with his curly hair framing a look of consternating, he replied, "We are going to need some luck or more information."

Our drinks had arrived, and I slowly sipped my Macallan, trying to savor the smooth, biting taste while cerebrally looking for light in the black tunnel before me. "Mike, the Chinese guy, Jin, seemed to be the bait that reeled in my buddies in Florida, and that occurred in the area around Ely, northwest of here. Do you think we might check out that area? Maybe we can find the guide he used up there to help us locate Jin. If we find Jin, he may lead us up the food chain—most importantly to those holding Emma, if she's still alive. I know this is out of my area of expertise, so tell me if I'm crazy."

Again, while creasing his forehead in thought, he replied, "I think that is the only way we can go now. I don't want to step into the middle of the "Kumbaya" moment my federal brethren are having, but I believe they might actually be happy with the assistance if we can provide it without the outside world seeing us on the nightly news with Lester Holt, Norah O Donnell, and David Muir all leading with the off-the-books, life-losing, property-destroying adventures of a heart surgeon and his sidekick from the state department. That would take us both into the unforgiving space inhabited by Bernie Madoff, Tonya Harding, Sam Bankman-Fried, and every other dazzling character that demands public scrutiny. If it does blow up, maybe they would label you the new Dr. Death, or at least Doc Holliday, and I'd be Wyatt Earp as we engage in the gunfight at the Ely corral—or hockey rink, whatever is most apropos. Ben, promise me you won't go all marine and get us in a gunfight? I know I brought the weapons, but those are for a show of authority as much as anything."

"Mike, just a hypothetical here, but what authority do you, as a State Department employee, enjoy in the state of Minnesota if we were to say, shoot a bad guy? The last I knew; the State Department was about international relations and reduction of tensions. I'm thinking that if we shoot a Chinese national while trying to do good in shutting down a drug ring or saving an American citizen, the consequences to your and my careers might be defined by a lot of time with lawyers, court appearances, and limited post event employment options. I also believe, though not certain, the Chinese government might make some loud pronouncements regarding the disregard for human life and rights in the gun-crazed America. I don't know; I'm just spit balling here."

The gleaming smile of my friend was both reassuring and unsettling. "Ben, again, I've seen you shoot. I am not particularly worried about you hitting someone intentionally. If it comes to shooting, I'll do it and ask our combined task force friends to take the fall. Some of them owe me, but I just don't think our investigation will take us there."

We were eating our meal, noting the quality of the steak being as good as anticipated. I asked the server if she knew where they sourced their meat. I was not surprised to learn it came from northwest Iowa. All were corn-fed and butchered locally. It was a little more expensive than the big commercial outfits, but the couple times they tried to switch, the clientele pitched a fit, she explained. So, for the last twenty years it had remained the same consistent quality. "It's hard to discount loyalty," I commented to her and Mike, the subtext to Mike being a thank-you. The server walked away, and I reengaged Mike on the region around Ely where I believed we would locate this Jin fellow or at least someone with a connection to him.

"Mike, on the plane coming up here I did a little research on Ely, trying to see about guides, the area, and perhaps how to approach it," I said.

He held up a hand and noted, "Given what my buddies shared, I, too, did a little research and have concluded this route of smuggling makes sense. There is about one hundred sixty miles of border with Canada in the Boundary Waters Canoe Area Wilderness. The BWCAW encompasses roughly one million acres, of which twenty percent is water. This wilderness abuts the Canadian equivalent, called the Quetico, to the north, and another national park, Voyageurs, to the west. Quetico provincial park is almost one point three million acres. The onsite authorities in the BWCAW are limited. Generally, a forest service employee will work with one from fish and wildlife, the first to manage the camping permits and the other to ensure compliance with fishing restrictions. The popular portage sites are the ones most frequently patrolled, and checks on the campers are made. There are approximately two hundred thousand visitors along the fifteen hundred miles of canoe routes and over two thousand campsites, according to my buddies and google. I think the ability to bring significant drugs into this country by this route is not to be ignored. Using a modified canoe built just for this route, a seventeen-foot canoe can carry one thousand one hundred sixty-five pounds of passengers and gear. If the gunnels were partially hollowed to allow storage of even a moderate amount of fentanyl powder, the math gets crazy. The wholesale price of fentanyl in large quantities is about one hundred thirty-nine dollars per gram. That would be about sixty-three thousand dollars per pound. You put roughly thirty pounds in the canoe, and you score just shy of two million bucks wholesale. If you have dealers working with small quantities, you could take your price from one hundred thirty-nine per gram to a thousand per gram. You are then looking at upward of seventeen million dollars for your effort. The risk of interdiction is low, and the money obscene. Five grams of fentanyl is enough to provide lethal doses to over two thousand people, they tell me. So, Ben, I think this problem you seem to have uncovered is a major issue, and thus the focused attention of all those alphabet guys on the federal payroll.

"I will admit the route is unusual, but the payoff even to small-time mules is big league. Getting the product out of the BWCAW is straightforward. By car, plane, train, or truck, the next stops are wherever the demand lies. Unfortunately, that takes in the entire lower forty-eight from there. I will admit we need to find the waypoint coming out of the Boundary Waters, and currently we have no real leads. That means we have a lot of real estate to explore. We're looking for a Jin in a haystack, so to speak." His toothy grin expressed his pleasure at his own joke. If he were a dad, I would have countered by deeming that a bad dad joke. Me being one, I had to applaud his effort.

I contemplated this information and the implications of the magnitude of our quest. "Well, I guess we head to Ely and see how the fishing is. I must be at Hazelton-Betty Ford tomorrow, and I'm unsure as to that time commitment," I noted.

"Yeah, I get it, and I think you stepping up for your partner is another sign of the kind of character you are and have. Take your time there. I'll head up to Ely in the a.m. and see if my buddies can point us in the right direction. If nothing else, I'll get us a guide, and we can have him or her show us the area and get a better sense of possibilities. If you are delayed, I'll fish to remove all the large trophies so as not to give you false hope in your infantile competitive mind of getting a bigger one or more. That, my friend, is just not possible for you." He flashed a shit-eating grin that I just couldn't help myself from liking.

Following dinner, we stepped into the bar for a nightcap and caught up on my family, his budding romance, recent travels, the status of the political climate, and then guns and shooting. "I grabbed you a Glock 17 knowing you have the gen-five at home," he stated. "I was able to score one here from the department armory. I have my Sig M17, so at least we can take comfort in knowing our weapons should the need arise."

My response was delivered with the understanding I wouldn't get an answer. "'The armory,'? you say. Is this an admission that you have been given an expanded job description with the State Department and I was unaware the State Department had an outpost in the foreign territory of Minnesota?" I said, bearing my own shit-eating grin.

"The State Department does indeed have an office in this wild and untamed wilderness; it has to satisfy the demand of its fine citizens to obtain passports allowing escape to the foreign sun-drenched beaches when it's thirty below here" came his response, as if he had been expecting my dumb-ass probe. "While that office does not have an armory glistening with all the latest in high-velocity projectile launchers, our brethren in the FBI and ATF next door do. Those good fellows allowed me to check out my toys using my Am Ex card as security." This was said so adroitly I wondered whether there was some fragment of truth in there.

"Well, I do appreciate the forethought and the effort in securing a gun I know. Since they are checked out with your library card, so to speak, and I'm not on a first-name basis with the special agent in charge here, why don't you keep them until I get to Ely. If I were to get stopped for some reason, I doubt my good looks would prove to be an impediment to a significant ticket and one law enforcement agency confiscating the property of another. Your 'loan a gun' buddies would probably charge your Am Ex for replacement. Which, as I think about it, would be damn funny."

We talked further, trying to seek some way to focus our broad search, but until we got up there and asked around, we were simply providing an excuse to enjoy the drink and disjointed conversation. We planned to speak over breakfast in the morning and then part ways, with the intention to meet up in Ely. Mike would try to get us two rooms at the Grand Ely Lodge. This, we had noted on the web page for area lodging, appeared convenient to everything and had a restaurant. It fit all the criteria.

I arose the next morning and caught Kay before she headed out the door for some school committee meetings. I reminded her I was going to be meeting with Tommy and his therapist today and then meeting Mike in Ely to try our luck fishing. While she understood the purpose of both was not strictly for pleasure, she encouraged me to have a good time and told me that she was on board with whatever we needed to do to help Tommy.

Mike and I met at a small diner with the ever-present fishing, hunting, and hiking motif. The walleye breakfast tacos were as good as advertised. The décor was cloaked in the seventies, with worn Formica countertops and plank floors. The option of espresso exposed the only thing out of character for this throwback of a diner. Our meal finished and plans made, we parted ways, he transporting firearms and I hoping for my friend's sobriety.

THIRTY-FOUR

THE SHORT DRIVE back to Center City allowed a brief respite for contemplation of my purpose. I felt nervous, with the experience being not unlike waiting for news from a doctor regarding test results or being summoned to the principal's office. The anticipation of bad news or consequences for a senior prank creates a hollowness filled with an emotional insecurity rolling in both the chest and stomach. While I knew I had not created Tommy's addictive behavior, I still felt somehow responsible. Would I be chastised for enabling or not being forceful about his obviously destructive tendencies? As friends, are we accountable to become the self-sacrificing moderators of reason when confronted with choices we ourselves have too often selected? This, despite cognitive awareness of their potential or real impact? How are the dynamics of human interaction guided when the perception of the same or similar experiences lead to widely differing interpretations of outcomes. Tommy and I trained together at the same time and place. We shared the same mentors and practiced in the same community from the same office. We had years of nearly identical day-to-day stresses, aspirations, and hopes. We shared professional decisions, and frequently personal ones. My relationship with this partner was a bond and yet here I was, summoned to account for myself and my buddy—or at least that is where my musings directed me. I was feeling my face bathed in the sharp, almost crystalline sun as I drove, the summer warmth rising quickly within me and around me, enveloping me as I flailed against my dragon of consuming responsibility. I knew my role in this visit was support, but perhaps my narcissistic doctor brain remained convinced that I could fix everybody and that to fail at that would be to fail myself. These thoughts confirmed my wife's frequent lamentations that we all needed therapy.

I then thought of myself and, on a larger scale, humanity. *Are the multiple aspects of personality or values we each carry within us our only true partners? They guide, chide, cajole, and generally control us minute to minute, day to day, until we have reached the end of this planetary existence. They have been with us since our brains were forming in utero and continued their maturation with us, side by side, until our twenties. Is it these "internal partners" we should pay more attention to? I would think obviously yes, but we truly need to know them first. Is this aligned with the 1 Corinthians verse "… so that there be no division in the body, but that its parts have equal concern for the other"? Have we not historically insisted our school curricula allow the teachers to meet all our internal partners and point out the pitfalls of giving free passage to those bad actors within us? While that may be the goal, I fear our educational system has been kneecapped by efforts to protect the discovery of our internal partners. We should learn in grade school to focus on those drivers of our destiny. God, how maudlin my musings.* Maybe Tommy's therapist would give us a group discount. I recognized I needed it, simply from this overindulgent oversimplification of the untold influences and chance encounters that establish our personal trajectories though life. I probably should be concerned!

I pulled into the parking lot of the campus-like grounds. By now, the green-leafed canopy surrounding the parking area offered a welcoming rustle of breeze captured in the netlike foliage of the oaks and aspens around the black pond of asphalt—the premier bastion of care and healing for those suffering from addiction. This multicentered enterprise in its current iteration resulted from the merger of the Betty Ford Center, cofounded by former first lady Betty Ford in 1982 outside Palm Springs, California, and its older namesake partner of the Hazelton Foundation. This arose from an old farmhouse in Center City, Minnesota, in 1949. Both were determined to provide a holistic, compassionate approach to a disease that few understood. The premise and success of their approach, I learned, was based on the twelve-step guidance of Bill W. and Dr. Bob, the founders of AA. There has been a lot of research, articles, and misinformation on addiction. The current understanding of the neuroscience came after I was through medical school and well into practice.

The brains of some individuals become activated by the chemical transmitters connecting the various centers and message lines. For the unfortunate few, this stimulation creates a need for repetitive excitation. The physical and psychological consequences manifest as the addiction. The brain centers must be satisfied. The potential for addiction is uniquely different between us. The sources of addiction are as varied as can be imagined. Sex, alcohol, porn, drugs, and gambling all can give the brain its neurochemical fix. The treatments that are successful may vary. For the drug addict, the addition of medicines acting as surrogate stimulants to the addictive center has revolutionized and enhanced care and success. For the alcoholic, there are some drugs that seem to blunt the desire and have been helpful, but the tenets of the AA founders, acknowledging a higher power and sharing the path to sobriety with others in an anonymous setting of conversational honesty and sharing of experiences, remain the bedrock approach of the foundation.

I walked toward the green-hued tunnel leading from the parking lot to the main door. This path had probably been traversed over the years by thousands hoping that entry into the building would result in a new life. The observant, shadowing, and whispering leaves and pines lining the walk seemed to offer protection to those seeking refuge, shielding against unwanted observers while speaking gently and encouragingly that help was near. This, I suspected, could be maintained in the harsh Minnesota winter by the evergreens backing the aspen and birches as reserve troops at the ready to protect the vulnerable. I was greeted by a pleasant, smiling middle-aged woman who seemed to exude a motherly demeanor and warmth that surely reenforced the resolution of those standing before her reception desk. "Good morning, how can I help you today?" was her greeting, delivered in a voice approaching angelic intonation. I found myself wanting to offer to help her. She was the perfect antidote to the AI-generated greetings of answering services or the frustrated, angry individual more commonly blocking your entrance to an appointment or at the department of motor vehicles. This woman should be cloned as the representative to all who engage in the public interface. Those ubiquitous satisfaction surveys that now follow every conceivable transaction, from parking lot use to brain surgery, would be rendered obsolete by the reproduction of this perfect greeter.

"Good morning. I'm looking for Dr. Moore. He is staying here, and I believe I have an appointment with him and one of his therapists. I'm Dr. Halle, one of his partners."

Her reply was "Certainly, I'll check the meeting room. Please have a seat. Can I get you coffee or perhaps some water doctor?"

"No thank you, I'm fine for now," I replied, not wanting to add to her burden of receptionist chores. Tommy emerged from a separate door, bearing the long absent grin and lively step I had known and appreciated all those years ago. If his mental transformation equaled this physical rejuvenation, I figured he must be about ready for discharge. The absence of alcohol, even for this relatively brief period, seemed to have brought the light back into his eyes.

I was gathered up in his bear hug and heard him say, "Thanks for being my friend, partner, and anchor. Getting here has saved my life." I was so relieved to find my friend literally glowing, with a newfound source of positive energy. This very brief exposure to the potential impact of his sobriety was the equivalent of the "born-again" transformation seen in the clips and movies of the tent revivals of earlier years or even broadcasts from the services of the current-day megachurches. Humans want to grasp the power they often find lacking within their core—the modern-day intra- and interpersonal corset that holds all the unsightly folds and blemishes of ourselves from honest interrogation.

"Tommy, I can't tell you how happy I am to see you and know you are getting healthy. Let's grab a cup of coffee, and we can catch up. I do have an appointment with your therapist at nine thirty, as I'm sure she told you. Also, here is the workout stuff you requested."

Taking his gym bag, accompanied by his ever-present grin, he stated, "Coffee is this way, and yes, I gave permission for Dr. Soma to extract and give any information she needs from you regarding me, your longtime fucked-up friend."

We proceeded to a quiet study or meditation room that gave the feeling of an outdoor space among the trees and shrubs of dogwood, hydrangeas, honeysuckle, and others I didn't recognize. The room had 270 degrees of its circumference windowed. Many of the windows were opened and screened, allowing the fragrances and sounds of Midwestern wooded summer to provide the backdrop to this island of reflection. Whoever designed the building and grounds understood the purpose of this space and the role of nature in magnifying the human experience.

Tommy gave a synopsis of his typical day. The calculated purpose to every waking hour was evident in the description of early rising, meditation, and group and individual sessions with therapists and speakers. There was free time for exercise, which for Tommy had led to a new passion for weightlifting. We chatted about his commitment to sobriety and his recognition of the detrimental impact of his behavior and addiction on to all those close to him. After we seemed to have exhausted his newly identified failings, we moved off the subject and talked about the practice and partners. This led to the heparin issue and the potential for other issues as well. I also revealed the absence of Emma beginning within a day of the driving incident. "Tommy, did you believe or know if Emma was involved in any of this?" I asked.

He paused and then offered, "She was telling me that night after we had a couple drinks that she and Kirk were obtaining a cheaper heparin and that they both were getting uncomfortable with making money from the deal. She said Kirk was going to talk to Howard in Pharmacy about formally switching to the cheaper product or changing distributors, as he felt the system was getting screwed by the pricing of the current distribution chain. The conversation continued in the car after we left, and I said the administration needed to know the details of the deal and the potential to save money but also get control over the pharmacy service. She was a little drunk and got mad that I would jeopardize her job. She tried to grab my arm to get my attention, and I, too, having had too much to drink, reflexively tried to get her off my arm and the steering wheel. That's when she got hit, and as you know, the ever-present boys in blue saw the act sans conversation leading to the act." He paused. "Why would she disappear? Do you think she ran off out of fear of the consequences to the heparin scam? That doesn't seem likely given her condo, her friends, and the fact she didn't organize this as near as I can tell."

I was then convinced a larger play was involved. Tommy's logic regarding Emma was solid. I then shared my thoughts about her being kidnapped to provide leverage over Kirk or Howard or both. I also now felt very strongly heparin was just a side deal to whomever was running this show. We were silent for a while, each lost in the various what-if scenarios. I looked at my watch and realized I needed to go find the office of Tommy's therapist. "Tommy, I've got my buddy Mike helping me look at all the factors, and when I leave here this morning I'm headed up to Ely, as we think there might be a connection to all of this there. I will call you if we find something."

I was again struck by Tommy's resolve to get better as he said, "Yeah, that's good. I'll be here a while yet, but if I can help, call me."

I found the office of Dr. Soma and was shown in after a couple of minutes. She was about five foot four, with blue eyes, short blond hair, sharp cheekbones, and a very disarming smile. I suspected she was homegrown stock and a powerful representative of the strong Scandinavian gene pool of the locals. "Dr. Halle, thanks for coming and agreeing to see me. We generally try to meet family members of our residents, but by Dr. Moore's description you are his family. So again, thanks. To put you at rest regarding our conversation, Dr. Moore has signed a waiver of confidentiality so we might share information." She spoke in both a professional and disarming tone.

"Tommy just gave me permission as well to answer your questions and provide whatever insight I might have regarding his addiction. So where to begin?" I asked.

We then spent the next hour together as I talked about my knowledge of his family and its dynamics; the pressure he always felt to exceed the expected and be better; and his drive to be the busiest, best, most liked, and most innovative, and all the while not to look that way. We discussed the pressures of medical school, residency, and then fellowship. We covered the competitive nature of every cardiac surgeon of our generation and the frequently repeated stories like Tommy's of seeking relief from the pressure through external validation, drugs, alcohol, sex, suicide, or, sadly, all the above. After an intellectual foray into the impact of the Covid pandemic to health-care workers and the apparent demeaning of science and scientists in the eye of the public and some politicians, we seemed to agree that the profound desire of our physicians and nurses to provide comfort, care, and healing was producing the stress of the unobtainable bar of perfection.

That bar of being perfect was being exacerbated by the litigious legal climate that existed, this quest for perfection diminishing professionalism. I was then startled by her question.

"Are you familiar with Aristotle? Have you read his works?"

I stammered a little, for obviously I knew of Aristotle, but my recollection of his writings was at best foggy, as I admitted.

"Aristotle believed that eudaemonia, or happiness and well-being was the greatest human achievement. Now, I'm paraphrasing from memory here, but he felt friendship to be one of the most indispensable requirements of life, and thus happiness and well-being. He described three types of friendship. The first, friendship of utility, where you are friends because you can provide something material to the other—or, in essence, a transactional relationship. The second kind of friendship is one based on pleasurable interactions like having a beer or the occasional dinner with buddies after work. The third friendship is the friendship of virtue. It is the relationship built over years of trust and interaction, the parties giving of themselves to make each other feel better. The act of giving is virtuous and does not require anything in return. I believe you are that third level of friend to Dr. Moore. It is refreshing and humbling to see that type of bond today. Society has abdicated personal interaction for social media and anonymous discourse. I'm afraid Aristotle would have to somehow create a new level of friendship that, sadly, would probably prohibit the attainment of well-being."

I was struck by this blond sage of relationships and the description of happiness and friendship delivered three centuries before the birth of Christ. I wished the conversation could continue, as I was now intrigued by the idea of motivation in my daily life and medical practice. I was again struck by my wife's words "We all could use therapy." I needed to pursue this when I got home.

"Before you leave, I want to quickly outline what Tommy's life will entail upon his return home. Given his arrest for DUI, the state board will allow him to keep his medical license only if he complies with the mandated random urine and drug screening for a period they will dictate, and the participation in an approved aftercare program. Fortunately, all the states recognize our programs and the success we have had with the compromised professionals. Our aftercare will involve Tommy attending group meetings of AA and finding a 'sponsor' that he can call or be mentored by. Those relationships vary, but it is critical that he find one and adhere to the sponsor's expectations. I will determine the need for ongoing psychological therapy depending on how he progresses here. While this may seem a bit onerous, it is a proven formula. I am asking you and the other partners to be aware of the stress he will feel on returning and allow some freedom for him to find a fulfilling life of sobriety. Your kindness and indulgence will make a tremendous difference in his life, far more than you already have."

I sat quiet for a minute as I absorbed these facts and my commitment and obligation as a friend and partner to help this man find his true self—not the self of substance-abused distortion, but the self that he deserved to be and the life he could choose to live. We parted in the entry to her office, I feeling somehow strengthened and, I suspect, she somehow more understanding of my friend's devolution into alcoholism. Tommy was in group therapy, so I left a note for him at the desk and headed to my car. I entered "Ely" in the navigation system and headed to the northern territories, at least in my head.

THIRTY-FIVE

I WAS APPROACHING I-35 north from Center City when my phone diverted me from listening to "The Hunter" by Doyle Bramhall. The title seemed apropos to my current quest of finding Emma or at least gathering some understanding of our pharmacy issue back in Florida. "This is Ben," I answered.

"Ben, it's Kirk. I just got a call from Emma. She told me I must get the missing drugs and money that Howard owes our new friends. She said she was in a canoe and couldn't talk. Then the line went dead."

"Canoe? New friends? Are you sure that's what she said?" I asked.

"Yeah, that's it exactly. When she said 'canoe,' I said, 'In a what?' But she talked right over me, and then she was gone."

"Kirk, do you have any idea about missing drugs and exactly where Howard fits in this?" I asked.

"No, but I'm headed to his office to see if I can get him to talk about it" was his response.

"Listen," I offered, "I think you should play dumb beyond the heparin issue. I'm afraid Howard may have been importing drugs beyond your deal. Why? I don't know. I do believe that if he is wrapped up in this, there is the potential for really bad consequences to anyone around him. I believe it best that he thinks you are only invested in the heparin fiasco. I wouldn't let him know about Emma. I'm going to run this by my fed buddy for his thoughts. It seems a little out of his area, but he knows some of the background here, and he may have gathered some intel that will give us a direction."

"Okay, I'll tread softly. This kidnaping of Emma and the missing money and drugs is shedding a whole new light on my ignorance. Are you sure we shouldn't let the local cops take this over?" He questioned.

"They seem to have not made any progress or even an effort in locating Emma, so I'm inclined to let them focus on the issues they know best: parking, lost dogs, speeding tickets. You know. If we don't make any progress up here, I'll give them a call." Was my reply that sounded more convincing than I felt.

"Okay, I'll let you know if Howard gives me anything. Ben, be careful, I think this is starting to have the stench of bad sushi."

"I will, and I appreciate the fish reference here in Minnesota. I'll talk to you soon." I clicked off.

The Bluetooth connection in the rental promptly told me another call was on. "'Ben, it's Mike. How are you, buddy?' was the reverberated greeting across the interior of the car thanks to the upgraded speakers in the SUV I had rented.

"I think I'm good. I met Tommy for a cup of coffee, and we caught up. I then spoke with one of his therapists. It convinced me we all need therapy. How about you, Mike, have you seen a therapist?"

"Yeah, my office has us all check in with an in-house shrink periodically. It's not really therapy; it's more like a quick check under the hood to try and avoid someone from going postal. Not that I think the competency level of those quacks is sufficient to recognize an impending disaster. To quote a John Sandford novel, I personally believe the shrinks are 'crazier than a cockroach in a crack house.' They probably don't believe what they hear and understand it even less. I guess now, as I say it out loud, I haven't had therapy but would probably benefit. I suspect my long string of noncommitted relationships stand as evidence of some sort of mental glitch. Then again, I may be leading the way to the new standard in relationship management: 'Be nice, be kind, be quick.'" He laughed.

"Your unmet psychological deficiencies aside, I got a call from Kirk a few minutes ago. He reported getting a call from our missing perfusionist, Emma, and she said she was in a canoe, which sounds crazy. In addition, she relayed that her captors wanted their drugs and money back. I know we felt this was something more than heparin, but this seems to confirm the theory. Finding a canoe with our girl in it seems impossible even if we have it narrowed down to this one state—which has ten thousand lakes, according to all the marketing material ever published by these Gopher-loving folks."

Mike's reply seemed loud, or perhaps its content was hitting the soft spot of my brain. "Ben, that seems to fit with the information I've been able to gather. As we discussed last night, this area is getting some attention. I spoke to my friends in the DEA and Homeland Security again this morning. Both shared their increasing concern about the Canadian–US border. They believe the cartels, Mexican and increasingly Chinese, are probing the northern border as a backdoor, so to speak. Much of the entire border is marginally monitored. The area around Ely and the BWCAW offer a tremendous natural enticement to those dirtbags. The patrolling is spotty, and in the summer the area has more than one hundred fifty thousand visitors. That makes blending in and being just another outdoor enthusiast easy. Then add the two thousand plus designated campsites and twelve hundred miles of canoe routes on this side of the border, plus even more to the north, and you have the easiest game of hide-and-seek possible. By law dating to Truman in 1949, aircraft aren't allowed to fly below four thousand feet over the wilderness. While maybe not helpful to smugglers, the nights are protected from light pollution through the designation of the BWCAW as an international dark sky sanctuary—one of thirteen in the US. In 2020, the BWCAW was designated as such. The entire five thousand five hundred twenty-five miles of US–Canadian border is pretty lax in terms of border security, but the one hundred plus miles of the BWCAW is, in essence, an honor system. If you have direct lake access to a Boundary Waters home without the need to go to a boat ramp, where there are volunteers or part-time verifiers that ask you where you are coming from, check your permits, et cetera. It's the private ingress and egress from the area that is giving the feds heartburn. While using this route in winter is more difficult it can be worth the effort from the return on the drugs. The place doesn't allow machines, but cross-country skis can provide access. I think your girl is probably on a direct-access lake, which limits our area of search, but we are going to need a little more refinement in our net tossing. When do you anticipate you will get to Ely?"

I looked at the navigation system and noted the "3:15 to destination" adorning my map. "I think around four if traffic isn't bad. Did you book a room?"

"Yeah, my local DEA contact got us into the Grand Ely Lodge that we mentioned yesterday. I took the liberty of getting you a room too. I know you won't sleep well without Kay, but I refuse to share a bed. You are just going to have to tough it out, big guy." He chortled.

"All right, but I think you are saving me from watching you embarrass yourself on the phone with the saccharine, over-the-top love cooing to your latest girlfriend. I'll meet you in the bar at five thirty. We can figure out how to reduce our area of search."

"See you there," Mike replied.

THIRTY-SIX

EMMA WAS AWAKENED by the footsteps of the pervert. Her internal clock told her it was an early arrival, and that provoked a mix of concern, hope, and fear. These last days, the routine had provided some comfort in the predictability. They had not improved the dietary fare being offered, but it was edible and seemingly indicated they wanted to keep her alive. They had not physically molested her, though she feared it was only a matter of time until they did. Her request to go down to the lake to bathe resulted in a bucket of water and a bar of soap being delivered by the perv. He put the bucket in the cabin while trying to stare through her shirt and then exited and locked the door. She was half expecting him to insist she bathe in front of him. She hurriedly washed her face, armpits, and crotch, and while trying to dry with her DEET-infused shirt, she listened for the return of her captor. She did not want to get caught with her pants down. She was grateful for the minor allowance of hygiene but realized she was still a mess by any standard. This early-morning variance from the routine was a first, and the significance or purpose set her imagination to warp speed. Unfortunately, the warp-speed thinking was more anxiety provoking than helpful. She needed to remain calm and be thoughtful in her response to this new situation.

Mr. Perv and Marathon Man both appeared, which was definitely out of the ordinary. They handed her a sandwich of peanut butter and jelly—a childhood favorite that for a second brought an internal smile of memory. She half looked for a glass of milk to complete the scene. "Eat it and come with us" was the simple order. This was accompanied by the very visible gun in Marathon Man's hand. They walked the path to the main cabin and then around the back, taking a path toward the lake. Waiting at the lakeside was the third man of the evil triumvirate. He was of medium build, with an angular face and a nose that had probably met a fist on more than one occasion. The dark hair was cut in a stylish, spiked, gel-enhanced fashion that remined her of a porcupine she had seen in the zoo. His dark eyes were focused on Emma—not in a sexual way, but more of a curious way. She noted the dressings on his left forearm and wrist. She realized then that his curiosity was probably piqued by the question "How the hell did this bitch end up cutting me?" With this realization, she was grateful those dark eyes weren't yet signaling a murderous anger. How long that would last was anybody's guess.

Two canoes were pulled up on the shore and were holding two paddles each and some bottles of water. She noted the absence of life jackets and thought maybe the coast guard or someone would stop them to check on their lack of prescribed safety equipment. Did canoes need such stuff? Was there a coast guard wherever this was? She was unsure. Being able to see that the width of the lake from where she stood was only a mile and a half or so, she doubted much of a presence of authorities. She knew that in California the forest service frequently encountered marijuana operations and acted as the cops. Maybe the forest service was around this area with the same mission statement as well.

They got into the canoes and paddled, she with the perv, and the other two—Marathon Man and Porcupine in the other. They stayed near the shore, where she noted the profound absence of other cabins. The paddling was distracting, and frankly it felt good to be moving her body with some rhythm and purpose. The lake was mirror glass smooth and clear such that she could see the rocky bottom in the slanted rays from the east-anchored sun. She guessed she was able to penetrate the depth to eight or perhaps ten feet. They had traveled maybe a mile in a generally northern direction when they gave her a cell phone that wasn't hers. The two canoes were being held gunnel to gunnel by her Asian crewmates. Marathon Man, who had always seemed to be the one in charge, said the phone was programmed to her friend Kirk's number, and when he answered she was to say precisely, "They want their drugs and the money back." He was pulling the gun from his hip holster and as an incentive added, "There is no reason for you to die today in this place where you will never be found. If you do as I say, and we can meet your friend to get what belongs to us, we don't care about you." It was that "We don't care about you" comment that said it all. "We don't care that you die when we get what we want" was the real meaning behind his statement. She was going to either need to make herself invaluable to these apparent representatives of the Han, Manchu, Hui or any of the other Chinese tribal populations. She noted that she was making a somewhat large leap in this ethnic assumption, but the little conversation she had overheard from the other canoe as they paddled seemed to be that of a Chinese dialect. Why they had paddled a mile to make a call probably had something to do with the nearest cell tower. Perhaps civilization and potential rescue were not that far off. "When your friend answers, say exactly what I told you. Have him repeat it and hang up. You will not say anything else. Do you understand?" he demanded.

"Yes" came the reply.

The call was made and strictly followed the script. *Now what?* she wondered. *If that was all they needed, do I have value? My plan of being invaluable needs to get some traction, but how?*

"Okay, I made the call, but why the need to do it from your canoe? Is there a purpose to this excursion other than providing me some exercise, which I want to say I appreciate?"

His reply was direct. "I wanted to see if you could help us in retrieving some product tomorrow, and you passed the test. Also, from our cabin we have no connection to the outside world. We could use a satellite phone, but as you may know, they are much easier to track and locate than the better cell phones of today. The GPS of the sat phone technology is like a beacon to the prying eyes of those we wish to avoid. Getting into this location gives us service with our encrypted phones. So, you see, this bit of fresh air for you was beneficial to us."

Emma looked at him and searched those dark, menacing eyes for signs of an impromptu life-ending plunge as he spoke. While processing the words, she was struck by her proposed involvement in the product retrieval. "So, you are telling me my paddling prowess has promoted me to some sort of waterborne drug mule?" she asked. His sickly, smiling reply of yes brought equal measures of hope for an opportunity to escape and fear of being around and in close proximity to these creeps longer. While they were still lingering on the quiet water, she metaphorically disturbed the surface with "Why do you need me to help you retrieve your product as you say? You obviously were doing this without my assistance before. What's changed?" The withering look led her to believe she had struck a personal nerve. She felt a chill, as if the water surrounding the tiny craft had lifted its collective cool depths to the surface to be brought by the breeze straight onto and up her shirt. The temperature of her aching, bruised body was dropping like a raindrop off a hat.

"Our associate was rendered disabled, as you Americans say, by your struggle when we went to your home in Florida," he offered. This was shocking, as she had not realized the struggle she must have made. If Porcupine Guy was a victim of her resistance and someone else was rendered disabled, she had to have been exceedingly lucky to only have been bruised and not far worse. She now understood there would be little compassion from this two-canoe navy if she didn't pull her weight in whatever was coming. The canoes separated and turned to return her to her cell. Reading her thoughts, Marathon Man said to her, "You will be expected to work tomorrow. If you don't, we have no use for you."

Rather bizarrely, Emma recalled a quote she attributed to Virgil, the Roman poet: "Carry on and preserve yourself for better times." Even if it wasn't the actual translation, she felt strengthened by this recollection and her interpretation. Tomorrow would bring a new opportunity, she was certain. She placed her paddle in the silent, calm water and pulled, visualizing with each stroke the moment she would be free from this nightmare.

THIRTY-SEVEN

I TOOK A left, taking the rental off Sheridan Street as directed by the map guidance, and a couple of turns later pulled into the parking lot of the Grand Ely Lodge. Its log construction reminded me of the home housing Ben, Adam, Hoss and Little Joe Cartwright of the on the TV show *Bonanza*. A large timbered porticoed entrance led to an expansive open area with chairs and couches constructed of the same hefty blond timber, all upholstered in moose- and bear-print cushions. To the left was a little commercial area selling Grand Ely Lodge and BWCAW shirts, jackets, sweats, and more. The preponderance of heavier-use clothing signaled the frequent mistaken summer visitor thinking that the June, July, and August climate here was like that of the southern latitudes. If these intrepid outdoor enthusiasts had checked the map latitudes, the recognition that Ely lies farther north than Toronto or Montreal would probably have induced them to pack a jacket that accompanied the bikinis and swim trunks. This fleeting thought brought a smile to my face, for I, too, had probably skimped on the warmer attire in my closet.

 I headed to the desk on the right side of the lobby and got checked into my room with a view of Shagawa Lake. The room was comfortable and in tune with the locale and purpose. The guests were generally there to fish (ice or open water), snowmobile, dogsled, or hunt. It was not a shopping or foodie hotbed of commerce. The king bed seemed comfortable as I lay back while looking at a map of the region I had gotten from the clerk in the lobby. It became immediately apparent that the innumerable lakes occupied as much surface area as exposed ground. The blue-paint-spattered blotches across the green forested puzzle pieces of road-deficient tracts seemed to invite an innate yearning to simply travel into this wilderness and be lost to civilization. I quickly understood the difficulties in finding individuals lost either by intent, accident, or poor judgment. This place was remote in body and spirit. The drive up from the Twin Cities deeper into the Superior National Forest provided glimpses of the dense intermixed conifers, aspens, birches, and shrub growth. A walk in the woods would be a difficult task off any trail, game or otherwise. I called Kay to check in and found I was personally missed; the kids were fine, and there had been nothing in the news about the potential heparin problem or the missing Emma. I was not sure how much longer that latter would remain unreported.

Five thirty found me sitting in the bar of the hotel, again admiring the consistent motif and the surprisingly comfortable bar stools. It was an obvious incentive to stay and drink longer. Mike appeared moments later as I gave my order for a Macallan on the rocks, and Mike added his Tito's with soda and a lime. This was expertly taken by a somewhat long-haired bartender and manager named Bob. We chatted with Bob for a minute. He was a longtime resident of Ely and seemed to know the locals and legends in equal measure. I cataloged Bob as a potential source of information going forward. After getting our drinks, we walked out onto the porch to discuss the latest in information. Mike informed me we were going to be joined by his new buddy Cliff Noble. Cliff was originally from the area but now worked with the DEA. He had recently been posted back here to get a handle on the extent and threat of drug trafficking from Canada. It was at this point we were joined by an imposing man with his large paw outstretched in greeting. Cliff was probably as stout as a local black bear, and after knowing him for less than five minutes I concluded he was as willing to protect his home turf as a mother bear protecting her cubs. His voice and manner displayed a possessive protection of his territory. The violation of the borders by those creating misery and death to his fellow citizens was as low as one could be on his scale of turpitude. His physical bulk of muscled arms draped alongside a barrel chest that supported a neck that seemed to have been cut short to add muscular width. Atop this marginally contained pressure cooker was a pleasant and engaging face. Given his aura of contained anger, I would have expected a boxer's nose with a scarred chin and eyebrows, but in complete contradistinction, a face of unblemished youth was retained in this forty-year-old soul. I wondered if his imposing body aborted the potential for physical harm from those who might chose to cross his path or value system. Cliff held in his left a Leinenkugel's beer that fit his man of the north wood's persona.

"Doc, it's good to meet cha" was Cliff's utterance as he pulled up a chair. "Mike told me you're a heart surgeon. Do you have to take the heart out to replace the valves and such, or is that just old wives yakkin'? My cousin had to have his aortic valve replaced when he was young, but I don't know if they took the heart out or not." I couldn't help but smile as I explained that we did not need to remove the heart to fix it. I asked how his cousin was doing, and he said he'd outgrown his "pig valve" and that when he had the new one put in, they used a mechanical valve that shouldn't wear out, but he was now on blood thinners. I explained the role and purpose of the blood thinners and the potential for problems related to them. The family medical problems addressed, we moved on to the problem of Emma's disappearance and the connection to Capital Medical in the Twin Cities and the apparent role of the Chinese middleman to the Ely area. I tried to give Cliff all the details I was aware of and my theory that other drugs were probably coming south with the tainted heparin that had started this whole thing. Cliff listened attentively and, when I finished, said, "Doc, I think you have struck gold with your theory because it fits with other information we have gathered over the last year. We believe that while the volume of drugs coming across from Canada is currently modest, the bad guys are refining their techniques, routes, and distribution from this area. I don't know if you are aware or Mike filled you in on our geographic and logistic challenges, but this is not a simple border like, say, the Rio Grande River in South Texas. The fluctuating line of the border through the Boundary Waters, the number of lakes in the boundary waters exceeding eleven hundred, the large number of seasonal visitors, the large number of private homes along the entrance lakes into the area, and the scarcity of agents to control the camping and fishing, let alone traffickers mingled among them—well, this is the wet dream of the criminal element among us."

Mike remained silent as I asked Cliff, "So, given the dimensions of the problem and what I would estimate to be a very lucrative return for the bad guys' efforts. How can we find them and Emma? It would seem they are almost invisible to all of us?"

Cliff's unblemished, unscarred face broke into a huge bear grin. "We cheat" was his answer. He went on to explain that with the cooperation of the Canadian authorities, the countries agreed to allow certain remote observational satellites that covered the area to be tasked to the areas of suspicious entry in the north and to the exit sites of the canoes in the south. This cooperation and those efforts had preceded the current situation by months. While it was only theoretic work thus far, by hourly analysis of the tracks of the canoes, a pretty good diagram was being created to direct the focused attention of him and his counterparts. They could readily determine the voyagers who were leisurely fishing and those that seemed to be more interested on speeding south This tracking was aided by the placement of an identifiable chip assigned to each permit issued for entrance to the area from both countries. Permit holders were to enter the area at designated points based on their permits. Length of stay was also prescribed by the permits. The chip technology was similar, in theory, to a transponder that provides airplane position and identification. They had not yet used this developing information for interdiction but were getting close to putting it in play. He believed our needs would give them the leeway to get the higher-ups to sign off on an actionable plan. The beauty of the system was that if we saw an unchipped canoe traipsing through the lakes, we could direct the authorities to check on them. This part assumed the authorities were in close enough proximity to get there. The reality was that the scarcity of agents might allow some to get through before we got there.

 I was encouraged by the efforts of the authorities but was dubious about being lucky enough to randomly stop a canoe that would be containing Emma. "I see how this will help in the overall drug traffic, but what about Emma and this guy Jin who seems to be heavily involved in all this?" I asked to both of my tablemates.

Mike answered, "Between Cliff and me, we have personally visited every guide or their boss here in Ely, as that was where your perfusionist, Kirk, spent those two fishing trips with Jin. We think we found the guide, and we are going to meet with him later tonight to get whatever details he might recall. "Great," I said. "Is he coming here?"

Cliff answered for the two of them. "Actually, there is a great restaurant in town called the Frisky Otter. We thought we would go and treat our guide/informant to their world-class lasagna. It might help him recall some details. If it doesn't, you will still have experienced some of the best lasagna outside of Italy, I swear."

We finished our drinks and signed the tab to my account and headed for the door.

THIRTY-EIGHT

THE RESTAURANT WAS toward the north end of town on the main street of Sheridan. The parking lot was large and crowded with cars and trucks. It struck me that these vehicles must come with a canoe as an option at time of purchase, for at least 85 percent of them caried a watercraft on the roof or in the bed of the truck. There was the occasional boat on a trailer, obediently following the all-wheel drive chariot to which it was attached. While not as plentiful, many of the transportation models were adorned with bikes to emphasize the culture of fitness and outdoor activities. This parking lot was the perfect chamber of commerce ideal of marketing to a society yearning for escape and increasingly accustomed to isolation thanks to the pandemic. We parked our naked unadorned vehicle and exited. Mike, too, had noticed the prevailing presence of watercraft and spoke: "No matter what this guy says, tonight we're putting a canoe on the roof of this thing before we do anything else in the morning—one, because we may need it, and two, because I feel like we stand out, and frankly, I'm embarrassed by our not keeping up with the Joneses." We entered the building and were struck by the enticing odors of good food enhanced by the herbs used to prepare them, along with the low, pleasant chatter of customers telling their own fish stories and encouraging their dining partners to outdo them by size, number, or human-versus-beast exploits. We were shown to a pleasant outdoor table with a small vase of what appeared to be native flowers, which truly set the tone of expectations regarding the upcoming meal Nicole, our server and co-owner of the place with her husband Mike, took our drink orders as Cliff noticed a tall, dark-haired six-foot-one-or-two man of about forty coming toward the table. It was difficult to accurately judge his age because of the weathered face that revealed prominent large almond eyes surrounded by raccoon rings of white, denoting his adherence to sunglasses, and a short black beard. Nicole had suggested we have their house special grasshopper. She explained that the typical drink of the same name in no way compared to this refreshing escape from the stress of life their customers walked through the door with. I was intrigued, and the four drinks arrived shortly. It was a good call on our part.

As Nicole departed the table to give us some time to talk and check the menu, Cliff introduced us to our guest. "Mike and doc, this is John Deer Davis." I immediately smiled and chided Cliff for falling in love with his dear at first sight. Cliff quickly disavowed any attraction to men as he tried to say "Deer" was John's real middle name. "It's the animal, not the tractor or emotional partner." It was amusing to watch Cliff so uncomfortable with the notion I had just prodded him with. I felt, even though I had just met both, Cliff and John Deer were going to be fun to be around.

Mike, piling on a bit, said, "Come on, Cliff, John is a good-looking guy; I can see the attraction."

It was really our good fortune that John Deer Davis immediately assumed character and joined in: "Cliff, honey, it's okay; we can talk about your feelings later. But just so you know, I will show you a good time."

None of us could contain our laughter as Cliff recognized how badly he was being played. I suspected this banter was going to be a part of the group going forward.

Three of us ordered the lasagna, while John Deer ordered the Italian beef sandwich. We shared a bottle of wine as we ate, and then coffee as we sought information from John Deer. "John," I asked while we were still eating, "there must be a story behind the 'Deer' in your name?"

"There is. I was the third child, and we were living a long way out in the sticks. There were no cell phones at the time, and the land lines were frequently interrupted by branches taking the lines down. My dad worked in one of the mines and was gone on long shifts and then followed work with a few beers with his buddies. He was a good guy but not the most consistent in his presence. Anyway, mom goes into labor and figures the best thing is to get to town or her sister's place about five miles down the road. Mom claims she was driving carefully but knew I was about to enter the world. She was debating her options when a deer darted from the edge of the road and ended up on the hood of the car. I guess the excitement of the crash induced a prompt arrival of me in the front seat of a '71 Ford pickup. Thank God for the bench seats. Well, Mom felt that since the last thing the deer saw was my birth, she should name me out of reverence to honor the animal. I really appreciated her not going with 'Bambi.' Now, that said, I guide hunters and take a deer every year with bow and arrow myself, but I do feel an allegiance to the animal. There was silence and more smiles at the table. At some level, I wished I had met John's mother. She had to be an interesting individual. Over the coffee, we got down to John and Jin and how that information could get us going.

"Tell us, if you don't mind, what you know about this Jin guy. I'm sure, but don't want to assume, Cliff told you our concern about his involvement in some drugs that got into our hospital system. We don't yet have any direct proof, but there appears to be a strong connection to him and what we have had to deal with."

John listened and answered thoughtfully. "I don't recall how he said he got my name ... perhaps from brochures I leave in the bait and tackle shops, or maybe online. It's been a couple years now, and at the time I was not sophisticated enough to track client referral sources. I do a better job now. I changed the name of my guide company and now generate a newsletter that goes to all the customers regarding open boundary water permits I have or fishing and hunting updates—that sort of thing. When Cliff called, I went back to see if I had heard from him after the last trip we took which was over a year ago. I had not, but it did remind me of the guy, Jin Wang. I took him out three or four times, and twice with a nice guy from Florida. I can't remember his name, sorry."

"Kirk?" I asked.

He smiled. "You are right; it was Kirk. I recall those two trips went pretty well. Got some nice walleye and a few northern. Kirk was a good fisherman, while Jin acted more like it was a duty or job—not something he felt natural or engaged with, if you know what I mean. The other trip I recall was with a big guy—I mean obese. It was tough to get him down in the boat. I recall he looked Asian, but that's about it. I'm sure they gave me a name, but again I'm sorry. I seem to think he said he worked in the cities. I have no idea doing what. I usually try to get my clients to meet me on the lake we will be fishing, but on that first trip with Jin, he asked if I would pick him up as he had car trouble or something. I was happy to do so, thinking a nice tip would reflect my Uber service. He gave me an address on the northwest side of Fall Lake. It was not far from a rustic cabin I have on a smaller lake. I spend whatever free time I can there or let friends and relatives use it. Fall Lake is a good fishing lake, and I offered to fish it that day instead of White Iron, but he said he was going to save Fall Lake for another trip. I believe he said the cabin belonged to someone else and he was renting for a few weeks. The interesting thing is, we never did fish Fall Lake, either that year or on any of the other trips. I assume he stayed at the same place, but I don't know."

Mike asked John whether he thought he could find the place on Fall Lake again. "I'm pretty sure," John replied. "I don't have much reason to be on the roads up there in summer, but I know of a hunting spot up off the Cloquet line that that was fairly close to the cabin."

"Is there anything else about Jin you can recall? Looks, build, tattoos, anything?" Mike asked.

John thought about it and said, "Yeah, I can describe him, but better yet, I should have a picture in my client album on my phone. I try to get one of all my clients with their catch. Let me look." He got out his iPhone and went to his library and albums and tried to get near the date he thought was around the time of the trip. After a few minutes and his showing us a couple of huge fish (by my standards), he said, "Here we go" and handed the phone to Mike and me. Kirk was standing next to a well-muscled middle-aged Asian man. He was probably five eleven or six feet, judging from Kirk's height. And he had what looked like a tattoo of a serpent on his left forearm. His face was plain, and his hair cut short. He seemed to exude a confidence rather than friendship, with a nearly sinister thin-lipped smile. It appeared that John was correct in identifying the fishing as a duty rather than a passion. That said, John was apparently a good guide, as they had a nice bunch of fish on the dock at their feet.

"Can you send that to me?" Mike asked, and he gave him his phone. Then he said, "Hell, just airdrop it to me now." The ether around us in the restaurant provided the transportation service without any of us feeling it. I couldn't wait for the human transporter of Star Trek to be available to us. We simply had to be digitized. Mike then asked how far out the cabin was from the Otter, where we sat.

"Probably twenty or thirty minutes," John said. "I don't mind if you want to go now—we have some light for another half hour or so—but I need to get back, as my wife has girls' night out and I need to watch the baby." We quickly settled with Nicole and gave the promise of a return. Cliff piled in with Mike and me, and we followed John out of town. I noted the Dorothy Molter "The Root Beer Lady" sign near the road and thought, *now this is America!*

As we headed toward the cabin, the warm, gentle breeze carried the pine-laden fragrance of the surrounding woods through the open windows. It provided mental reset to remind me I was no longer in the balmy, humid environment of Southwest Florida. I was a universe away currently. Cliff explained that the Cloquet line was originally a railroad track line that was used to take timber from the Superior Forest. Spur lines off the track allowed the log haulers to get the timber out onto the lake, where it was then floated down to the mills for cutting. He added, "If you are on the lake, you will see a couple sites with a line of old track pilings out in the water where the timber was offloaded." I found this piece of history intriguing. With the waning golden light highlighting the low whispering leaves of the forest on either side of the car, Cliff brought us back to the task at hand. "When we have identified the cabin of interest, I'll have my guys run the ownership tax rolls. Also check the electrical use, et cetera. Most of these places are seasonal, but increasingly they are being winterized or rebuilt for year-round use. As if on cue, John had pulled over to the entrance of a drive. There was a locked gate of some substance in place, and what looked to be a security camera mounted high on a pole about ten yards down the drive. The drive circled to the left and was lost in the tree cover. John said, "I'm pretty sure this is the place, though I don't recall a gate. I guess it could have been open, and I simply ignored it." While there should have been a fire number, none appeared to have been posted. John then added, "I need to head back to town, if that's all right." We all concurred.

"John, do you have to guide tomorrow?" I asked.

"To be honest, I had a trip but gave it to one of my buddies after talking to Cliff. He thought we might want to check one or two of the lakes around here."

"Thanks for that. We will do some work tonight, and I'll call you first thing in the morning," I said. The two vehicles headed back to town and the lodge for us, home for John.

As we drove, Mike stated some thought-provoking considerations. "We need to see if this cabin is currently occupied—and if so, by whom. If occupied, we need to get eyes on and perhaps in the cabin. We need to see how the chip tracking trial is looking for the lakes around here. While Fall Lake looks promising, there are others that could be as useful. I suspect more than one route is being trialed. We need to know who owns Capital Medical. We need to get some Google Earth shots of this portion of the lake. We need to find your girl Emma. Am I missing anything?"

"Finding ownership of the cabin and Capital Medical should be easy, and if they are one and the same, our worry meter can be raised a notch."

Mike said he would try to get his fed buddies on some of this now but quickly found we had no cell service. "I think I'll get us a couple of sat phones if this is going to be an operational area," he said.

Cliff quickly added that he could requisition a couple out of the local DEA office in Virginia, Minnesota and have them delivered first thing in the morning. Mike then reminded me we needed to add some canoe accoutrement to our rental vehicle. "Absolutely," I said. "I think we will be up some creek, and I want both a canoe and paddle. We may need some camping gear, depending on what intelligence comes back tonight and in the morning. I'm sure John can advise on those issues."

Twenty minutes later, we brought our SUV to a rest in the lodge parking lot. I was beat and said I would meet the guys in the lobby at six-thirty for coffee and planning. Bob and Cliff both said they were going to make their respective calls and have a beer. "See you in the morning," I said, heading up the stairs to the second floor.

THIRTY-NINE

EMMA WAS QUICKLY awake as the footsteps approached her one-room compound. She was standing and looking at the limited dark sky through the window. It was chilly, and she was considering wrapping the scratchy blanket about her but nixed the idea. She wanted free hands and did not want to give the slightest impression of weakness to these assholes. The door opened after the perv had managed to master the process of getting the padlock released. He didn't command her to step back but simply handed her a microwaved burrito. *I'd better use the outhouse; it's going to be a long day.* The idea of this grande-sized, gas-inducing bean-and-cheese lump residing in her belly for the next however many hours was competing with her need for energy. Well, energy it would be. If this fart-producing fare was the option, so be it, and she hoped her emissions would prove toxic to the guy in the canoe with her. She managed to eat most of it on the trail to the outhouse. The sky was not yet revealing any eastern inflammation, and the stars were brilliantly shimmering fireflies against a black satin backdrop. Then she noted, low on the horizon as she rounded a curve in the path, the fluctuating flame like shards and strobes of light escaping the margin of earth and sky.

The low, undulating, and wavering purples were trying to envelop the gold and green sea of light beneath their royal drape. This was the northern lights she had heard about from friends and books. It was a spectacular reminder of the magnificence of the universe and how truly insignificant she was in it. She was unsure whether this represented a good or bad omen. The day would provide, as all days do, the unfolding plan before her. The sight was so mesmerizing that both she and the perv stood transfixed by the vision and recognition that power was contained not by humans but by forces and energies generally unseen. The excitation of atmospheric electrons seemed to provide something similar yet profoundly personal in these two happenstance observers. The heavens were hinting at the unknown with this brief exposure to the immense power held elsewhere far from these spectators. They blithely traipsed to an unheard drumbeat carrying them from mundane lives to collisions of fate. Perhaps that was the secret destiny of all humans, now made more apparent than usual by this glimpse at grandeur and its comparison to a life loop of blunted, emotionally encrusted living. *Yes, today is going to be different,* Emma thought. The heavens were showing her.

The outhouse duties completed, and her mouth rinsed with a bottle of water, Emma and her three captors walked the path to the lake. The men each carried a backpack or duffel, and they had given Emma a backpack of her own. Its contents were not particularly heavy, so she assumed the trip was of a short duration. There was a cooler pack carried by Marathon Man. All four had been given a canteen of water. At least that's what they claimed. They approached the two canoes pulled up on the rocky shore and pushed them partially into the water before loading them. There were footfalls on the path coming from the cabin, and Emma turned to see a distinctive man in jeans and blue denim shirt with a red vest coat. He appeared to be roughly forty years old. He was tall, at slightly over six feet, and trim. There was no denying his ancestorial origins as Asian. Emma wondered if these guys were all related or simply the local chapter of the Chow Mein Mafia. He spoke quietly to Mullet Man and then addressed Emma. "If you work hard as part of this team, I believe I can see a way for you to leave these woods alive and perhaps with a little money. If you are a burden to my friends, I will have no trouble allowing them to enjoy the delights of your body and then offering your remains to the animals of these great forests. Do you understand?"

While she intended to sound defiant, the noise that dribbled from her lips was a simple yes. He looked at her with such searing, penetrating eyes that she almost felt violated standing on the rocky shore. The light breeze pushing the lapping water across the stones at her feet reminded her to stay focused and believe. It was all she had now. This she understood. The two canoes were then pushed off and headed into the slapping water that gave a metronomic cadence as it struck the sides of her craft. The aurora had vanished, and the slightest of pale pink touched the eastern sky, trying to return the fireflies of the night back beneath the blue blanket of the day sky. It was faith to believe they would return tonight to gaze upon this waterborne band of nomadic voyagers.

FORTY

I WAS STILL on Eastern time and thus was awake long before common sense would dictate. On typical workdays I arose at five, so in the time zone of today I was wide awake at four. I felt a jog would help me organize my thoughts, so there I was when Mile-a-Minute Mike passed me on his return to the lodge as I was getting ready to turn at a mile and a half out. I tried to push myself a little, and graciously Mike slowed to allow me to catch up. "So, I think we will get out to that cabin this morning and try to get inside if it's confirmed it is related to Jin and what's been going on," he offered. I found the fact he wasn't gasping to talk irritating, God, I was pathetic. "Sounds like a somewhat criminal plan" I managed to get out, accompanied by the last little spittle that I had retained in my parched throat. "I hope your relationship with the local gendarme has been bolstered by more than your looks."

"We will be covered. If we identify a connection with your drugs and these guys and this location, warrants will follow, even if we perhaps are early in the execution," he chattily offered.

"So, considering I'm about to require CPR and you, my friend, look as fresh as if you just jogged ten yards, I have to ask. What's up?" I got out between gasps.

"I got in shape this last year. I ran the Marine Corp Marathon and then in March the Napa Valley Marathon. Nice venue and refreshments!"

"Okay, now it's evident I'm competing in a different class. I'm relegated to the slow, fat, and special needs category, as in 'needs oxygen.' But I accept your challenge even though you didn't vocalize it." I saw we were only a quarter mile from the lodge parking lot and sprinted, or at least in my mind I was sprinting. Mike was by me in short order and said, "See you in the dining room in thirty minutes. You are buying." I wasn't sure my cardiac recovery would be normalized in thirty minutes.

I found Mike and Cliff in the dining room with coffee before them and one waiting for me. "I understand you put the local EMS on high alert this morning," said Cliff. "I didn't realize they provided way station coverage for a quarter-mile jog. I'll have to remember that."

"Well, I at least got out there, and I will admit style points were absent, but it was a beginning. I just didn't realize the altitude difference between here and Florida. Must be like ten thousand feet," I said, watching my dining companions nearly spit out their coffee. "What have we learned over night?" I asked, wanting to get off the subject of my bruised macho ego.

Cliff was quick to begin. "My associates in DC told me this morning that the cabin we identified last night with John and Capital Medical, the distributor, are owned by the same entity—Qiang Holdings. They are trying to get more information, but it seems the cabin was purchased with an adjacent piece of property four years ago. Capital Medical was purchased from a company called White and Sons about the same time as the cabin. It appears both were cash deals. My guys are trying to track down the prior owners of both entities to see if they have any further communication or information from the Qiang group. The Virginia, Minnesota, agent that delivered the sat phones this a.m. also grabbed some night vision eyewear for us—two PVS-14 monocular units. I asked him to go out and observe the cabin this a.m. until we decide on a plan of approach."

Mike stated, "I think we might want to approach the cabin from the water and the land simultaneously. I suspect we all agree and are confident the drug business and this cabin are related. I believe we can get a federal warrant if Cliff's guys know a friendly judge. There is obvious increased sensitivity to Chinese-based drug producers and cartel activity, so it should be an easy sell for the warrant. I'm hoping to get an update on boat traffic from the satellite geeks this morning. Thanks, Cliff." He then added, "I think we should probably get prepared to go on the water, whether it's to get to the cabin or follow them if they are moving. Ben, I strongly feel we will find your perfusionist out there with them. There would be no advantage to having her holed up somewhere and not knowing what it is they think she has on them. I think that if she isn't in the Capital Medical facility down in the cities, she is up here. Cliff, do you think any differently?"

Contemplating, Cliff replied, "No, I think we should be ready to move on the cabin at least. If the girl wasn't in play, I might say we sit tight, but I'm afraid delay may prove costly to her. The hope and assumption are that she is still alive. We know she made the call on their demands, but who knows now."

I chimed in. "You guys are the experts in this, so I defer, but Cliff's logic makes sense to me. I say let's at least clear the cabin."

Mike remained quiet but nodded his agreement, or at least he didn't disagree.

Cliff said he was going to try and get an update from the computer guys and call John Deer Davis to ask for his assistance in guiding us if we needed it going into the Boundary Waters. He would also get a list of supplies he thought we might need. He suggested we go arrange for rentals and then hang loose until he had a list from John and the information from the geeks monitoring the waters. This all seemed like a long shot, but at least we were moving. Five minutes later, Cliff called as we were heading for an outfitter. "John is in. He will pick up some food for a couple of days but said to rent the lightweight Kevlar canoes and lightweight sleeping bags, and, importantly, buy plenty of mosquito repellent."

"Got it," Mike replied into the phone as we headed down Sheridan St. The emphasis on "lightweight" did not go unnoticed as we drove. "I'm thinking we have some portage work ahead of us if the dudes aren't in the cabin," I noted, thinking of how gassed I was on the morning jog.

Mike smiled. "Buck up, buttercup, I'll carry your ass if need be. Just don't make me do all the paddling."

"Deal," I said. Mike then reminded me we had the guns in the back of his rental. "We will be armed, and you will not shoot me by mistake. If you do, this carry-your-ass deal is off the table."

"If I shoot you, it's because you needed to be shot, and I will be the final arbiter of that decision. So mind your manners," I said, knowing my bluster was probably weaker than a spiked lemonade at a Mormon church social. Ten minutes later, we pulled into a generous parking lot with an outdoor display of kayaks and canoes that would seemingly provide transportation to the entire fifth fleet. I was feeling watercraft envy as I looked at the shiny, sleek above-the-surface torpedoes that would deliver the equivalent of the minor league marine expeditionary force, as portrayed by us, the four comrades now committed to rescue and drug interdiction. Would wonders never cease?

FORTY-ONE

EMMA HAD TRIED to get a conversation going with Marathon Man, who shared her canoe. They were about twenty-five yards behind the other canoe and were well past their second portage since striking out in the dark. The light was brilliantly reflected off the water. A fact Emma was well aware of as she had no sunglasses to protect her eyes. The breeze seemed to have picked up. It didn't seem to matter whether they veered right or left following the lakeshore; the wind apparently was stuck directly on their bow adding to the eye and muscle fatigue and making the day all that more tiresome. During the portages, Emma had tried to envision an escape scenario. The intellectual exercise was short circuited by the effort needed to haul the canoe and pack over the rocky terrain. It seemed she was required to give more than fifty percent of the muscle of the two-man team.

She assumed it was about noon when they pulled ashore, and she was offered a couple of granola bars and some water. The three men sat on some rocks and, while not welcoming her in the circle of trust, the conversation didn't force her out. Little was said among them until Marathon Man stated, "Our boss and his partners want to know what you did with the drugs."

Emma looked at each of the men and tried to see if she understood. "We used the drugs for the heart surgery patients. That's why we bought it from you guys."

Mullet Man smiled with a face approaching a snarl. "Not the heparin. The fentanyl. We know it didn't make it out of your storage area. The people who sold it to you want their money or the drugs. If not that, they want your life and your partner's. We are on our way to gather more product, and by the time we get back, our associates in Florida will either have the things they desire, or they will have ended your partner's life, as we will end yours. I thought sharing this truth with you might prompt you to remember where you put our drugs or money. You should think on this as we continue our journey."

The chill Emma now experienced was from both the words just spoken and the falling temperature and rising breeze on the water. She needed to be planning an escape or attack, but simply sitting in the canoe like a dumbass wasn't going to be helpful.

They pushed the two canoes into the water and resumed the trek. Once again Emma was convinced the headway was being hampered by the elements, not the least of which was her less-than-best stroking effort. It seemed to her the longer they took going somewhere, the better off she might be. Over the next two hours, she was yelled at to pick up her pace with threats to put ashore and beat her. With each of these, she would pull a little harder for a while and then again slack off. She was expecting a physical rebuke soon but would not make herself try to speed up their arrival to whatever awaited. As she tried to devise a plan other than stalling, she noted the small white caps cresting the increasing waves. They were pushing toward them from the left side of the canoe bow, which she then recalled was the port side of a boat. *And isn't a canoe a boat?* she thought. The breeze was now pushing fine spray off the rolling and increasingly large waves, and they were coming in a quicker pace as the thumping, rolling, and sliding of the canoe took each of the water thrust punches. The other canoe was slowing in the water, and the two men ensconced in there were talking and gazing to the northwest. Emma followed their gaze, and as she had seen earlier, the sky was filling near the horizon with a charcoal-colored pillow of menace. The tops of this adornment looked alive in undulating motion. There seemed to be a vertical push and then an eastern expansion, as if chocolate milk were being spilled from the heavens and coming across the intersection of earth and sky to catch whatever and whoever was beneath.

It was about then the flashes began penetrating the mixture, creating a green-and-white transitory window into the cauldron. The temporal juxtaposition of this display from the nocturnal aurora she had witnessed was disorienting. The light show was followed by the rumble of warning. This show was not going to remain in the upper atmosphere. The warning was from the skies and was telling them to heed this announcement. She was convinced the Chinese gang of three heard it as well as she.

The two canoes were now adjacent to each other and rocking with the increasing urgency the water imparted with each thump of its aquatic fist. They were beginning to wear the spray on their faces like a lotion of roughly applied face cream that would never soak in. The falling temperature could have passed for a cold cloth administered to reduce swelling and anxiety. The latter, unfortunately, was rising with the wind among the stalled smugglers of the Boundary Waters. Within the next short minutes, sitting in the canoes on open water would be a potentially fatal flaw in their quest for drug-fueled money. The slow paddling effort Emma had been displaying a few minutes earlier was now replaced with a vigorous rapid-paced pull that reflected the sudden fear that was shared among the canoe occupants. Emma was recalling the news stories of derecho winds, tornadoes, microbursts, and waterspouts. All these labeled destructive storm forces were suddenly real in her mind. This reality was confirmed with nearby flashes of lightning and the resounding booms of thunder that were felt in her throbbing chest as she strained to get the canoe to shore. The dark now enveloped them as pellets of rain struck their exposed skin. Small pellets of ice were now mixed into the composition of the stormy brew. The strobe-like light of the lightning cast eerie glimpses of the nearing rocky shore. The bow of her canoe struck a boulder and was pushed to the right, where another boulder was struck and pushed them to the left. The painful onslaught of wind-driven elements of water in its visible forms of liquid and ice allowed their eyes eyes to be only partially open. It was enough to see and feel the canoe rise and twist along its length with the shifting of the packs and the water in the vessel bottom. The delayed reactions of the occupants contributing to the weight displacement and the canoe now on it's side

Emma and Marathon Man were in the water, and it was chilly but felt warmer than the ice-bearing air above the water. While a good swimmer, Emma realized she was dogpaddling trying to get oriented and find the canoe. Her hands slapped a hard object, only to find it the slick side of a rock. She was gasping and felt panic adding to the weight of her clothes and shoes. She then heard the guttural grunts of her canoe-mate behind her and the splashing as he grasped for her in a desperate effort to keep his head above the waves and off the rocks. As his hand found the neckline of her shirt, her feet found the bottom of the rocky lakebed. His desperate pull brought her head under the water, and her tenuous foot perch was lost. She then reacted from adrenaline-fueled survival mode as her head came up. She swung with all her strength at the dark, panicked eyes. They had now forgotten their fixation on her tits and saw her as a life preserver that was within his grasp. The blow, while glancing at best, was effective in allowing her the freedom to again stand, albeit without confidence or stability. "Stand up, you dumbass!" she yelled. She could see the overturned canoe over his bobbing head and tried to step toward it. He thought she was reaching for him and again reached and clutched her arm, with the same results as earlier. They were now both beneath the waves, and Emma felt the rocky bottom with her feet and then her knees as they struck larger, barely submerged boulders. The pain in her lungs from their inability to obtain air and the increasing alarm-bell pain that was now rising from her right knee competed for attention in her brain. Her one focused thought was that she needed to get to the surface and drown her tormentor, or at least escape his grasp. If she could accomplish that, she felt, her survival would follow.

She felt the disturbed water at her back as her panicked assailant was groping for any part of her he could clutch. She summoned a memory from childhood and crouched down to the bottom, aided by her heavy wet clothing, and tried to place her feet beneath her on some sort of semistable ledge. Her feet found a small platform, and she looked up through the water. While the darkness of the storm prevented any substantial light from penetrating the water, the increased darkness of the body above her provided a target. She pushed upward with all her might, the pain in her right knee exploding simultaneously with the flexing of her arms and tightening of her fists as she struck violently into the neck and chin of Marathon Man. There was an audible gasp within the turbulent water, and she felt the sensation of her fists compressing cartilage into spine. Her head came out of the water as she desperately tried to refill her lungs. She treaded water a few seconds and then found the bottom again with her feet. She was aware that her right knee was unstable, and the sensation of additional warmth against the cool water elicited the image of blood from a damaged joint despite the fact she wasn't yet seeing anything below the water and blowing rain and spray above it limited her view of the surroundings to just a couple feet. She felt the bump of a hand to her back, though it was not the motion of desperation and in fact was not purposeful. She reached behind her back and pulled the hand toward the shallows where she stood. She tried to turn herself, but the pain and instability prevented her from a full pivot. She innately knew that the hand she held was now attached to a dead man undulating with her in the waves in a macabre dance that was neither choreographed nor sought by either party. Yet they moved in synchrony from the unseen force of nature and circumstance.

FORTY-TWO

JOHN JOINED CLIFF, Mike, and me as we looked at canoes to rent. With his advice, we settled on a seventeen-foot Kevlar fiber model. He repeated several times that we should not run into objects with this watercraft, nor load it on land and drag it into the water, as we were likely to damage the epoxy and resin binding and degrade the canoe if we did so. This was reinforced by the manager of the outfitters reminding us of the loss of our damage deposit. While I tried to portray the air of a competent canoeist, the comments of Mike and Cliff—such as my marine service involving amphibious assault vehicles powered by diesel engines, and that my soft surgical hands had yet to be calloused in any manual endeavor—all seemed to minimize my persona in the eyes of the recreational manager of the year, as proudly displayed on the wall over the checkout counter, this complete with his smiling mugshot. Hell, he probably had T-shirts made for family and friends with that picture.

We finally got checked out of the store with supplies that felt indispensable, and a credit card charge to confirm the same. Cliff then took a call stating the agent watching the cabin had reported no activity and he would stay there until we arrived to go onto the property. After a brief conversation, we decided that Mike and I would approach the place from the water. We had identified a boat launch site adjacent to the Fall Lake Campground and a short paddle across the lake to the cabin. Cliff and the agent from Virginia, Minnesota, and John would come to the cabin by car and on foot. We would call to synchronize our arrival and before going ashore, and we would try to observe the cabin and grounds from the water. We went our separate ways, Mike and I headed to the boat launch, and Cliff and John heading up the road. Thirty minutes later, we were putting the canoe into the water. After grabbing the paddles out of the back end, Mike slipped the two handguns into his pack. This he placed in the canoe as I pulled the SUV up the ramp to a parking spot. We had decided to leave the rest of the gear in the back of the truck until we had confirmed the need to go into the Boundary waters.

We quickly got into a smooth, coordinated rhythm and were making good time across the lake. We both noted the darkening horizon and understood the implications for the probable delay of heading into the BWCAW if we decided it was necessary after the cabin visit. We reached the shore adjacent to the cabin and tried to look like a couple of water enthusiasts. Mike then commented that we should have thrown our fishing poles in the canoe but somehow, he had overlooked that bit of subterfuge. "Jeez, Mike, I thought you were the professional spy here. This is more like an Inspector Clouseau caper. At least we aren't wearing dress slacks and shirts. We could try to shoot a fish with our pistols to not look conspicuous," I said, laughing. "And by the way, you haven't commented on the smooth and professional manner we've managed this canoe."

"I'll concede your ability to push the water with your wooden stick there, but if there is any shooting, it will be me shooting you for being annoying," he retorted with a chuckle. "Now grab the binoculars out of the bag and let's see if there is anyone around."

A few minutes later, after glassing both the cabin and grounds albeit with some lapses due to the thick tree cover near the structures, we were convinced that no one was moving or visible. That did not mean no one was home.

"I'll call Cliff and tell him we are headed ashore." Stated Mike.

The call completed; Mike handed up the Glock for me to have. I secured it, and we paddled to a small sandy patch along the shore of the property. We stepped into the shallows with our newly purchased water shoes on and walked the waterline, trying to maintain focus on the cabin and surroundings. I was listening for any audible warning or threatening noises. This immediately returned me to my marine training of recon patrol.

Cliff and his fellow agent approached from the entrance road and left John to watch their backs and to call if someone showed up. They slowly approached the cabin and noticed a shed off in the trees about forty to fifty yards. Cliff said he would go to check it out and left the other agent to continue to watch the main cabin. Cliff slowly approached the shed from the rear and through some underbrush and noted the wild blueberries and a few red raspberries. He observed the sloping roof and absence of windows in the back. Making his way around the corner, he saw the open slant window high on the wall toward the front of the cabin. He stopped and listened. There was no noise from inside. He stepped around the corner onto a path in the front. The door was unlocked, but a lock was in place. He slowly pushed the door open and noted the smell of an unemptied urine bucket. The remainder of the place was remarkable only for a blanket on a thin mattress. Someone had been using this place recently. He strongly suspected it was the missing Florida girl.

Cliff exited the shed and took the path toward the cabin. He spotted the other agent and signaled him to head toward the cabin from his location. He scanned the grounds below, but the view of the water was limited. He did not see me or Mike. Taking his time and trying to match the methodical pace of his agent counterpart, he saw the path swinging to the left slightly, and the water below now came into view. He glimpsed Mike in the trees and understood Mike had seen him as well. A few more minutes and the four men converged on the cabin from the four sides, with myself coming in opposite Cliff and Mike coming up from the lakeside. No words were spoken, and with a hand signal Cliff indicated he would go in if Mike would cover and come too. Nods were exchanged, and Cliff stepped up the two steps to the door. He mouthed, "One, two, three," and he swung the door open and entered. He quickly moved left, and Mike, on his hip, swung right. Within a couple of minutes, the cabin was cleared.

They looked for anything that might provide evidence and pulled a shipping invoice from the trash that had Capitol Medical letterhead. The invoice was to a Canadian company with a Vancouver address. Cliff said, "I think this might be their counterpart, but we will need to quietly check. He took photo of the receipt and replaced it. The shed has been used, and I believe it was most likely your missing perfusionist was in it. It looks like they are on the move. The question is where to, and by what route and how long ago." As he concluded his summary, the sky quickly darkened, and a loud clap of thunder shook the structure. John appeared in the door and announced the impending arrival of a big storm, this information having come to him from his fishing and outfitter guide buddies. With this development, Cliff and

John suggested Mike and I remain in the cabin out of the storm and then retrieve the canoe after it passed. They would return to the truck and try to get any more information on the storm and to talk with the geeks monitoring the lake traffic here and further north over the last twelve hours. It was unlikely the girl and her captors had been gone for more than that—or at least that was the hope.

As Cliff and John dashed out the door for the truck, it started to rain and blow with increasing ferocity. "I guess timing is everything. I'm glad we weren't caught out on the water in this. I'm afraid for those that were," Mike noted. The wind was now providing a howl to accompany the pounding of rain and the metallic chatter of small hailstones striking the roof. The air was alive with energy, but the sunlight could no longer color the canvas of their surroundings with anything other than various shades of gray. They were deprived of visibility both literally and figuratively as to where to go next.

FORTY-THREE

THE WAVES HELPED propel Emma to the shoreline, though she was unsure whether it was an island or mainland. It didn't really matter; she was out of the water. But the incessant rain continued, though with less ferocity—and fortunately without the hail. The wind was persistent and blowing steady and hard against this respite of rocky shore she had landed upon. She took a few labored steps inland and tried to get behind a large rock beneath a pine tree. It was minimal protection, but it was something. She examined her knee and the long laceration that ran from above her kneecap to well below it. More disturbing was the lack of a smooth surface to the kneecap. In its place was a rather sharp, angled defect of the bone. She recognized this as a fracture line. She also recalled some anatomy—that the extension of the lower leg occurred by way of the tendonous attachments above and below this fractured patella. When she tried to extend her leg, it did so with tremendous pain and very weakly. She suspected the fracture was not quite complete in dividing the kneecap into separate fragments. At least not yet. Walking was not a reasonable option without crutches, and walking on this rocky shore with crutches seemed about as likely as her walking on water. That was what she needed now—a godlike intervention: a short stride across the water to shelter and safety.

She remained behind her rock—and, as much as practical, beneath it—to maintain some body heat and stay out of the elements. She was unsure as to how long this cocooning lasted but after probably an hour or two, the grayness began to lift, revealing the green of the trees and the browns, reds, and yellows of the stones at her feet. She tried to lean against her backstop boulder as she rose, using her left leg to elevate her from the crouch. Just the passive movement of the right leg brought tears to her eyes. Perhaps some of that may have been due to self-pity and emotional exhaustion, though there was no denying or minimizing the pain. She got turned to face the water and saw the body of Marathon Man rocking against the stones in the shallows The inverted canoe was down the shoreline perhaps twenty yards There was a pack bobbing next to it. To cover the twenty yards seemed an impossible task, and to not try seemed a surrender to this whole shitty saga. She needed a crutch, and for that she turned with difficulty toward the trees. There must have been thousands of usable crutches waiting in the forest. She simply needed to go find one—the caveat being it had to be close by.

FORTY-FOUR

MIKE AND I sat in the cabin and discussed the storm and its implications for us and those we were trying to pursue. We concluded that if nothing else, they would be forced, like us, to seek shelter. Their head start, if they were on the water, might be reduced if we got going and knew where to go. They should have had no idea they were being sought by us, and thus their sense of urgency would be less than ours. But again, in what direction and by what means should we be trying to catch these guys? Thus far our evidence had been as much intuition and mental gymnastics as it had been based on facts. We were, however, strengthening the ties of Capital Medical to this cabin and seemingly to our drug problem in Florida, and, we hoped, to the presence or absence of Emma. The evidence thus far was so flimsy a fart would have shattered the pedestal we had rested it upon.

As the sun broke through the clouds, Cliff came through the door. "I got ahold of our geek guys, and they reviewed the last twelve hours of water traffic in the area. It looks like two canoes left here about three this a.m. and headed toward the first portage up the lake. Interestingly, about the same time, a truck left here and headed south. They lost it going toward Virginia. That is forty miles or so from town. They are trying to re capture the canoe traffic now with the storm over. They are basing their search on estimating the distance they covered before the storm. They said the canoes were moving with purpose but did not seem to be sprinting to a destination. I guess we can hope that assumption is correct."

Mike and I looked at each other, then at Cliff. "Cliff, tell us your thoughts and we will go with it. Tracking and getting the bad guys is your wheelhouse," I stated.

Cliff answered without hesitation. "We all head out now. We need John to guide, and we have the sat phones to keep in touch with our overwatches. I'll get somebody to track down any vehicles associated with this place, Capital Medical, or Jin. If they find one, we will put out an alert. In the meantime, I'll get twenty-four-seven surveillance of Capital Medical. If they show up there, great." We all agreed, and as Cliff made some calls, Mike and I helped get his canoe from his truck with the supplies he had and carried it down to the lake. Twenty minutes later, we were out on the water as the last of the rain shower dissipated, leaving the air cooled and fresh. The soft splash-pull-drip noise of the paddles seemed to mesmerize me. If the circumstances were different, this would have been a cool adventure. The adventure part at the moment was being emphasized by the presence of the Glock on my hip. That just wasn't cool.

The two canoes expeditiously crossed the lake and retrieved the stored gear Mike and I had left in the truck at the landing. A quick inventory seemed to confirm we were ready, but our food was probably limited to a few days unless supplemented by fish.

Cliff and John then led us northwest to the first portage. We efficiently unloaded the canoes and distributed the items in roughly equal measure, though I had the sense that Mike and John took on heavier loads. John had brought along his .30-06 rifle with 220 grain bullets and kept it in a waterproof soft case.

This he had laid within reach as he paddled, and he repacked it the same following the short portage. Cliff informed us that his geek buddies had identified one of the canoes now on the water, but the other was not visible to them. The moving vessel appeared to be slowly working the shoreline about twenty miles ahead of us. We were quickly speculating as to the reason, and the first conclusion was that the storm had separated the voyagers, and we were being given an opportunity to make up some time and distance. The cool experience of being on the water was devolving into a tryout for a position on a college crew team. My recent fitness deterioration was being exposed with every one of my pathetically labored strokes. Apparently, robust, bulging biceps were not enhanced by the daily needle manipulations of the cardiac surgery I performed. I reminded myself that my lack of physical endurance was compensated for by intellectual endurance. I could think beyond any cardiac surgical challenge, dammit. However, if getting to the patient involved rowing or running, they might as well grab a Bible and cram for the final. The returning sun following the storm was welcome but easily provoked the sweating accompanying our labors. We were making a strong effort to make up time and shorten the distance to our presumed prey.

FORTY-FIVE

EMMA SEARCHED THE ground around herself and found a couple of stout branches of about eighteen inches, these having resulted from the storm's denuding of the trees nearby. She struggled to pull the small sprouting branches and buds from the selected pieces and then took off her soaked shirt and bra. She used the bra to wrap the sticks along the sides of her knee. She found that when it was wrapped tightly, she could then use the clasp of the bra to hold the whole wrapped splint in position. She found a smaller stick to slide beneath the splint. If twisted, it would create an even tighter wrap. She took care not to create a blood-halting tourniquet with the risk of permanent damage or limb loss. She tried to wring the water from her shirt before putting it back on, but the chill of it against her skin was shocking. She looked skyward and became aware of the golden glow and reflected pinks from the setting sun. The calming water of the lake was now trying to mirror the early evening sky, as if to apologize for the torment of earlier. This celestial offering of a serene surface and still air, the wistful appearance of heavenly order in the subdued light and gentle *lap, lap, lap* of the water on the rocks—it was as if a cruel joke were now regretted by God. "Just kidding, Emma," she could hear God whisper in her ear. "This little misunderstanding should not alter your believing in my benevolence." Well, she had to admit her belief was being tested.

With the knee splinted and the sun rapidly approaching its collision with the horizon, Emma hobbled toward the trees in search of a crutch. After fifteen very painful minutes, she found a reasonable option. It was about the right length and had a natural bend at the end that probably had been a branch prior to the storm. It now created a facsimile of the top of a crutch for her armpit. She tried it for a few steps and was turning toward the lake. She saw the canoe containing the perv and Mullet Man coming around the corner. She sat down roughly, eliciting a grunt of pain. She was behind a fallen tree, and some of the bigger rocks on the shoreline prevented their direct vision of her. She was certain they would see the body of Marathon Man, which was now lying like driftwood on the rocky shore. The dark bottom of the overturned canoe might not be readily visible in the twilight and could be mistaken for rocks. She strained to hear their voices and was torn between getting their attention or being quiet She heard Mullet Man say it was getting too dark and the shore was too rocky here. They decided to reverse their course and return to a better spot to beach their canoe and resume their search in the morning. They mentioned something about the time to meet the product, but she could not catch anything else.

 She watched them glide around the point they had come from. Emma slowly got herself up. The throbbing pain took her breath away whenever she stepped wrong or tried to put her lower leg out front to balance. She let some tears run down her face but would not break down. She would show them. She would get through this. The sliver of moon would not offer light to check out the body of her dead castaway companion, and it was too dangerous with her limited mobility to try and grope around in the dark. The need for some protection now struck her. There were bears, wolves, and who knew what else here that might want to make a meal of her or her deceased captor. She hobbled back to the woods excruciatingly slowly, wincing with every step. She couldn't go far, but she needed some shelter for protection and a few rocks for a potential encounter with those wishing her harm, either human or animal.

FORTY-SIX

MIKE AND I tried to answer the unanswerable questions: Are those canoes our suspects? Are they armed? Is Emma with them? Is Emma alive? Is it better to follow or confront? The most pressing question was that of whether to camp for the night or press on. This was answered unanimously among the four of us. We would press on. John knew the waters and felt the next portage could be managed in the dark with our headlamps. We had a few more minutes of daylight, and the next portage was an hour away, according to John. We all grunted our agreement, with my grunt perhaps being more guttural than the others, as my body felt it deserved a vocal contribution due to its being asked to provide a largely atrophied set of muscles to the effort. Paddle on we did, the headlamps of the four of us creating a gliding, steady beam across the dark water. This unnatural luminescence, accompanied by the soft splashes of the paddles and the rhythmic breathing of my companions, was as calming and tranquilizing as a namaskar or the sound of silence in mediation. I realized I was in complete synchrony with not only Mike, who sat a few feet behind me, but also Cliff and John in the adjacent canoe, and myself. I had unconsciously moved from awareness and discomfort of myself to feeling a universal sense of peace and belonging here on the water. If only it would last.

We reached the next portage and got the packs transferred to land prior to beaching the canoes as we were advised, given our Kevlar-constructed craft. The portage was roughly a half mile.

The path was generally smooth and of a gentle slope except for roughly twenty or thirty yards. This was steep and required some care in carrying the gear and canoes in the dark. On reaching the next lake, we took a quick break, and Cliff checked in with the eye-in-the-sky guys who were assisting this posse. As he did so, I tried to describe to Mike and John the Zen-like moment I had experienced. To their credit, they said they understood and had had similar experiences as well. I admitted that it was so near orgasmic that I was anxious to get back on the water and try to recapture it. They both cautioned that it may or may not occur but that being open to it was half the battle.

Cliff then stepped back to our group and reported that the single canoe had beached and there was a small fire nearby. The important fact was that this was not a designated camping site, thus giving more credibility to this being at least some of the group we wanted. We finished our energy bars and drinks, relieved ourselves, and then got the canoes in the water and reloaded. John estimated we would be near the beached canoe in a few hours, at least while still dark. But without a precise location, he told us, we would need to stay offshore and be exceedingly quiet, as the ability of sound to carry over water would not be our friend. We all agreed, and Cliff said he would check in with the geeks in a couple of hours to see whether the fire was still burning and to confirm some GPS coordinates for us to focus on.

We set off, and I tried to recapture my previous meditation aura but found I was completely distracted and focused on the confrontation I was expecting, hoping that Emma would be found sitting around the campfire. Our pace was steady and set by John. He was obviously at home in the situation of being on the water and in search of prey. Cliff seemed to mimic John's attitude, or perhaps that was his natural self—calm, focused, and intent on bringing down the enemy. I could relate to that from my marine training, and the ability to focus on a single task for hours on end defined the brains of most cardiac surgeons I knew. Mike seemed to be constantly altering the situation and its impact on our approach and potential success. This was exhibited in the whispered questions he put to me: "Are you ready to shoot from the canoe, to kill another? Will you be able to swim under fire? Swim and shoot?" I recognized these as being rhetorical but also that he was running through scenarios and options out loud. I simply answered and tried to plan accordingly. I believed I would do what was called for but fervently hoped it would be a simple walk up to them and a "You are under arrest," and we would all live happily ever after.

A couple hours later, we halted our stroking and could barely make out the darker mass sitting upon the water as land. Cliff made his call by sat phone and confirmed yet again the coordinates we were headed toward. The fire was only a slight glow on the image as reported by the geeks. Someone was getting some sleep, it appeared. We looked at the map John had pulled out as we held the canoes together. He checked our location on his titanium Fenix 7X pro watch and announced we would be off their location in a little over ninety minutes without pushing it. That would get us there an hour before sunup and allow us to set up prior to daylight. He showed us the spot on the map where the fire was located. It appeared to be in a little bay on an island of perhaps a quarter mile by a half mile. He said we should try to get as close as possible to them before going ashore, as bushwhacking through the islands under growth would be noisy and tough unless we wanted to take hours doing it. We all looked at the map and, after a minute, concurred. We identified a point around the corner of the little bay from them where two of us would land. The other two would stay in their canoe and converge from water as the others did on land. We would try to coordinate our arrival by sat phone signal. It was decided Cliff and John would land their canoe and Mike and I would be the coast guard.

FORTY-SEVEN

EMMA TRIED TO close her eyes, but her old nemeses, the mosquitoes from hell, had no mercy in their swarming attack on exposed skin as the sun set, the biting being exacerbated by the tormenting buzzing about her hair, eyes, and ears. There was no position or motion she could find to lessen the onslaught. The tears of pain, frustration, and fear only seemed to embolden this airborne version of black death. The blackness matched the depression of her psyche and to some extent the little saucer-like space she was ensconced in on the ground. Despite the darkness now cloaking her, she felt exposed and was regretting not getting the attention of the two surviving captors. At least there would have been some human to share a little of this physical misery with. She then caught herself and realized they probably were going to kill her any way. At least being here alone, they wouldn't be around to enjoy her final moments. She had to stop this pathetic pity party. There would be something good when the sun came up, and she could try to salvage some stuff from the shore and perhaps the canoe. First on the list was some water.

She was unsure of how much time had passed, as the moon seemed to have barely moved across the sky between the branches of the tree. While the stars did their best in covering the blanket of black with tiny sequined dots, they provided no real illumination, and she had no celestial knowledge of the names of the clusters. She remembered reading they were called "asterisms," those named groupings such as the big dipper. Their movement and position relative to hers on earth had never been of importance. Where the North Star was located may as well have been Midtown Manhattan. It had just not been relevant. She thought that if she survived, she might try to learn something about the subject. Hell, the sailors of the 1500s used them to cruise the oceans; how hard could it be? Such distracting thinking allowed her to ignore the knee pain and the itching at least temporarily.

She was trying to think of the names of some of the asterisms when she heard a soft splash on the nearby shore. She listened intently and gripped a stone in readiness to ward off the animal, whatever it was. She also had next to her a slightly pointed stick. If the encounter came to that, she would at least try to make the son of a bitch sorry it met her. There was another slight splash and the movement of stones beneath the weight of a paw. *God, it must be a bear*, she thought. She remained absolutely still, her breathing shallow but rapid. The night chill was now seemingly ice cold as she broke into a sweat. Her stare into the blackness provided no information. She could see no movement, and no other sound was made.

She then heard steps to her right. They were only brief, but she definitely heard the rustle of branches and the slight crack of fallen ones from the storm. *Is this how bears sneak up on their prey?* Maybe it was a large wolf. She considered screaming to scare it, but her voice was lost somewhere in the midst of her fear. The next thing she heard was the low voice, almost a whisper, from a man: "Don't move. I have a gun, and it's pointed at you."

Her lost voice returned, equal parts exhaustion, relief, and wonder. The whispered response of "I can't move much; I think I broke my kneecap. Who are you?"

"My name is John," he said, slowly but remarkably making his way through the dark. "You must be Emma." He reached her at the same time the tears and sobs erupted from her battered body. After holding her for a minute to allow her to compose herself, he explained he was with three other guys, one being Dr. Ben Halle. With that news, another brief gasp of relief and tears followed.

"Where are they? There are two guys who were holding me still out there, and there is a dead guy in the water near a capsized canoe. I think I killed him or he drowned, but he is dead. Can we get going before they come back?" She was saying all of this and realized he was trying to get her to lower her voice.

"I don't want to turn a light on here, because we think the two other guys you mentioned are just through the trees on the edge of the water. I'm going to leave you here for a bit and go see if I can find them." She now noted the rifle slung over his shoulder. "My partner is a little farther down and moving toward them as well."

She then saw he was looking through a complex-appearing monocle that she immediately understood was a night-vision system. "Is that how you saw me?" she whispered.

He nodded and said they had also seen the overturned canoe in the water and the dead guy on the rocks. She asked for some water, but he had come ashore without any. "Sit tight," he said, peering at her in the dark. "The sun will be up in an hour and when it is light enough, we are going to get the other two guys. Will you be okay for now?"

"Yeah," she whispered. "Please don't forget to come back."

He squeezed her arm and then crept silently into the undergrowth.

FORTY-EIGHT

MIKE AND I held our canoe offshore and observed Cliff and John make their way to the rocky beach. With the night-vision device, we could see them step out of their canoe and examine something at the water's edge. We then saw Cliff raise an arm and make a slashing motion across his neck—the implication being that someone was dead in the water. God, I hoped it wasn't Emma, but I felt that was the most likely situation. A short time later, they saw John and Cliff diverge up the shoreline and move into the trees. Once out of sight from our mates, Mike and I slowly stroked toward the point and held the canoe just short of rounding it. The eastern sky was showing just the faintest glow. The stars began to lessen in intensity along the curtain of earth and sky. Against that rising fire, the stars held no strength to continue their nocturnal display. They would quickly retreat behind the blue, like a set change of a stage play, to await their nightly encore of spotlighting the heavens and earth, to the delight of humanity. We had planned to come around the point when the sun would be rising into the little bay. The geek guys had pinpointed the campfire as situated just around the point and almost facing east—probably in response to the storm winds that had come hard from the west the day before. We figured their attention would be to the rising sun, which would give us a few more minutes to close from the water and for Cliff and John to come at their backs.

The awakening dawn was accompanied by the report of a gunshot. *Shit,* I thought. *Who shot that?* With the presumed element of surprise and a coordinated approach now apparently relocated to the trash bin, joining most other plans of warfare and engagement, we stroked hard to come around the point just a few yards off the rocks. With Mike in the stern paddling, he whispered to me to get my gun into firing position. This I had already begun, and I was systematically searching the edge of the woods for any threats. The smoldering remnants of the campfire were less than fifteen yards from our bow. Beyond it I saw a man looking to the trees, holding a gun, and a little farther past him was another, also armed but turning his gaze toward the rising sun. The harsh reflection off the water seemed to be impeding his ability to immediately see us. Mike commanded, "Drop your weapon," now aiming his at the figure facing us. The placid water allowed the canoe to provide a stable shooting platform. This was confirmed when the man facing the trees turned and raised his gun to shoulder height. The loud, unmuffled crack from Mike's gun was followed by the gun-toting shoulder in question rocking violently back and the gun and the hand that held it both dropping to the side of the challenger. His scream of pain was enough for his buddy to drop his weapon and raise his hands. This was quickly followed by Cliff and Mike exiting the trees and going to each of the men.

Cliff produced some zip ties from his cargo pants and had the uninjured one held with his hands behind him. We were now getting our canoe secured on the rocky shore, and I went to the wounded perpetrator. He was Asian in appearance, but his vocabulary of English vulgarity seemed complete. His right shoulder was going to require an orthopedic surgeon to put the joint back together. The good news for him was that the axillary artery that travels beneath the joint was intact and functioning, as indicated by the presence of a pulse at his wrist and a lack of major arterial bleeding. The nerves may have been bruised by the proximity to the bullet's trajectory and perhaps some bone shards, but they, too, most likely would allow function. I bandaged the entrance and exit wounds using a first aid kit from our canoe, and we made a sling for his arm. As I worked on him, Cliff informed us of finding Emma, scared but okay in the woods, with a possible knee fracture. The report also included the presence of the dead body and overturned canoe. As soon as this information was shared, Cliff and John returned to the woods to get Emma and the canoe they had beached in the dark.

A short while later, we were all standing or sitting on the shoreline and discussing the next steps. Emma had given us all a great hug and had a difficult time in containing her tears. These were interrupted by silence, then some swear words directed at her captors, and then the cycle repeated over again. We got the story of her kidnapping and her vague memory of the bloody encounter at her condo. She now believed the blood was from one of her captors following the scuffle. She then explained the purchase of the cheap heparin and the hope that she and Kirk would make a little money on the discount difference. I questioned her on the role of Howard in Pharmacy. She thought at first that he was not aware of the dealings but that he had become more attentive and secretive about Kirk or her retrieving the drugs from the delivery dock. She had concluded her kidnapping was because these guys and Howard were getting narcotics delivered to the hospital, and then Howard got them to some local guys, but that part was speculation. She believed the canoe trip they were taking was to pick up more drugs and try to use them as leverage to motivate Howard to find the last shipment or the money from it. They seemed to think Kirk was involved in the missing merchandise, thus the call they had her make to him. She didn't believe Kirk was aware of the narcotics and assumed that Howard had probably panicked with the scrutiny surrounding the bad heparin. She had been unaware of the heparin issue until my current questions. She hadn't been to work that day because of her bruised face, and then she was kidnapped.

This led us to the discussion of what we were to do next. Fortunately, our uninjured prisoner was listening and offered some help and information if we would maybe let him go. Cliff, representing the legal authority, said only a judge could agree to that; but given the need for action, he would try to make the case for leniency to the judge and prosecutor. He was quick to add that the guy was in deep trouble because someone had died in the commission of the felony, and that the penalty for death involving a kidnapping and use of a gun could be life without parole. Whether Cliff was being truthful I was unsure, but it got the attention of the man Emma had dubbed "the perv."

The perv, aided with the grunts of affirmation from his erstwhile partner, the newly labeled "one-armed Jack," told us they were to meet the shipment of drugs later this morning at an island farther up the Boundary Waters. John produced a map, and after some back-and-forth, we identified the transfer site. Given the time, we would not be able to mobilize a formal interdiction team. The people that were to be met were expecting two canoes and four Chinese nationals. We decided that Emma's perv would come along as the bow rider in the first canoe, and One-Armed Jack in the second. We would travel with three canoes and stop short of the island for Emma to stay back in the third canoe. John, with his dark hair and weathered face, could perhaps pass as Asian until up close, so he would be in the lead canoe with the perv. Cliff would be lying in the bottom of that canoe, and I would be in the bottom of the second with One-Armed Jack, leaving Mike to do the paddling. All the visible occupants would wear baseball caps and sunglasses. According to Mr. Perv, we should be meeting two canoes and four guys. *Let's hope so*, I thought.

Cliff had used the sat phone to give the location of the overturned canoe and dead body to the US authorities. We had pulled the body of the deceased ashore and covered it with rocks to minimize animal attention. Cliff also gave the location of the planned meet. A call back several minutes later informed him there were three canoes that were most likely headed to that location. He asked that they keep him updated, and we expected to be at the meeting site within two hours. I turned to Perv and asked, "How do you transport enough cocaine in the canoes?"

He smiled and said, "It's fentanyl powder and pills." He stepped over to one of their canoes and directed me to turn back the edge of the gunnel. I did, and it opened on a hinge, revealing a spacious chamber between the external hull and the interior bed of the canoe. The whole thing was virtually undetectable unless the canoe was closely scrutinized. The space along either side could conceal millions of dollars' worth of the drug—enough to overdose thousands. This was scary.

FORTY-NINE

THE THREE CANOES paddled in the direction dictated by John. The sky contained random cotton balls drifting slowly from unseen currents toward the east. The temperature was quickly rising, suggesting a warm day in store. The slight ripples across the lake surface were there only to break the reflected blue from above. The occasional shadow of the dangling clouds highlighted the brilliance of prism colors adjacent to their shadowed margins and rendered dark with the passage of the surface disturbance. The distance seemed inconsequential at this point. We had retrieved Emma; we now understood the role of Kirk and Howard, and I was awakened to the hidden threat being delivered to my community's doorstep—literally delivered to the doorstep of the very institution at which I spent hour upon hour trying to help the populace, one and all. The most revolting realization was the irony of treating the unfortunate individuals with infected heart valves due to intravenous drug use, and those drugs coming to them from the hospital loading dock. I realized my anger was rising exponentially as I was forcing the paddle with a vengeance through the water.

About twenty minutes from our destination, we pulled our watery caravan into a protected inlet. We gave Emma a sat phone and the contact number to Cliff's geek buddies. We reviewed the rules for the perv and One-Armed Jack. They were simple. If they tried to warn their friends of what was up, Cliff or I would shoot them first. It sounded threatening enough, but I was unsure whether I could shoot an unarmed man. I hoped not to find out.

They acknowledged the rules and said there was no preordained signal allowing us to get close to them. They again stated they were unsure as to why there were three canoes with the other guys.

Fifteen minutes later, we were nearing the site provided by GPS and the geeks. There were two canoes visible on the shore, according to Mike. Being in the bottom of the canoe, I couldn't see anything. Mike whispered that John and Cliff were about ten to fifteen yards in front of us and off our bow to the right. Mike muttered, "Perp at twelve o'clock on shore. Appears armed." The paddling in both canoes came to a stop, and the guy on shore yelled to One-Armed Jack, "What happened to you?"

To Jack's credit, he said, "Slipped getting out of the canoe last night and fucked up my arm."

The response was worrisome. "Who you got pullin' that paddle? Don't know about strangers. Where's your crew, man?"

The interrogator was staring dumbly at us as Mike said, "There are two guys to the left, short of the trees. I think there must be a couple more we aren't seeing." Just then he added, "One more guy to the far right." As this was coming out of his mouth, the guy in front raised the gun in his hand. Before he got a shot off, Cliff took him out from the other canoe. I heard the high buzz of bullets passing too close to my rising head. I felt the vibration of the canoe and the exhalation of air as the perv took a round in the chest. Mike and I both rolled right into the water, and the motionless body of the perv joined us as we sought some cover with the canoe. I came up focused on the shooters to our left. Coming from behind the stern, I saw one guy on his knees trying to catch sight of Mike. I put three quick shots toward the center mass of his body. He started to stand but then fell, face-planting onto the rocks. I saw the other of the shooters in this quadrant stepping behind a tree. The two shots from Mike's gun caught the tree hugger in the groin or ass, depending on your perspective. There was a bloodcurdling, almost womanlike scream from him as he grabbed his crotch. Cliff and John had taken out the other visible shooter to the right. It was probably unfair in that both shooters focused and fired on the bad guy simultaneously. The result appeared to be instant death.

We were all in the water, including One-Armed Jack. He was trying to get himself to the shore, but it's tough not to do a circle when you only have one arm and the other is acting as an unwanted tiller. Cliff barked, "I count four down. I wonder where canoe number three is?" We waited for a bit, hearing only the splashing of poor Jack trying to exit the lake. Mike and I got behind our canoe and, using it for cover, maneuvered along the lake shore standing on the bottom. Cliff and John did the same going in the opposite direction. We had traveled perhaps a hundred yards and saw a canoe up near the woods. We both stared intently into the trees and underbrush. It was very subtle, but the flash of metal in the broken light of the forest floor betrayed the site of the remaining drug mules.

"Did you see that?" I asked.

"Yea." Mike answered.

"Any ideas on how to get this 'OK Corral' thing over?" I asked. I was unsure whether I made this smartass comment because I was scared or because I was stupid.

"Well, I think we tell them to give up. They're surrounded."

"Okay, that might work. We shoot the guy if he refuses?" I asked.

"I guess so. I'm not anxious to go charging up this beach of rocks. If we don't get shot, we break an ankle."

"Agreed. Go ahead," I said.

Mike then pronounced in his best government voice, "You on the shore. Come out with your hands up. We have you surrounded."

This nicely delivered request was met with a quick succession of six shots toward us, some striking the canoe, others the water before and aft of us. We both popped from either end of the bullet-punctured canoe and concentrated fire on the place of the glinting gun. A soft curse and crashing branches followed. We pushed the canoe to shore and each came out as quickly as possible, diverging from the craft to the trees. We crouched and slowly worked our way to the nesting site of the bad guy. There was a body with a headshot that had stopped any further response in this life. Next to the body was a trail of blood into the woods. "If my math is correct, I think there probably is just one guy left, and he's wounded," noted Mike.

"As a part-time marine, I'm not eager to follow the wounded guy into the woods. I think he would have the advantage of an ambush," I stated. "Let's check our canoe and, if need be, borrow theirs. One of us goes to get Cliff and John and figure what's next. One of us stays here. The wounded guy may want to come back and claim a canoe to get out of here."

Our canoe, while not quite colander-esque, had several holes below the waterline. The mule canoe was pristine. Before borrowing it, I quickly checked the gunnels for dope. As anticipated, many plastic bags containing powder were attached to strings dropping into the frame. The weight of one string was perhaps a couple of pounds. The street value of the haul was hard to comprehend.

I easily paddled back to Cliff, John, and One-Armed Jack. I explained the situation, and we then collected all the canoes. We heard pleas for help a few yards down the shore and turned to see a man desperately clutching his groin and moaning loudly as he sank to his knees, his hands full of blood; a badly distorted scrotal sack missing at least one, if not both, of the family jewels; and a viciously shortened manhood. I approached and confirmed that he was going to need major urologic reconstruction. Unfortunately for him, it appeared the bullet had traversed his rectum before exiting. His surgery would require a colostomy and repair of the holes in the poop chute. His recovery was not guaranteed.

After trying to get some dressings in place and getting the guy in a canoe and lying down, we made our way back to Mike's location. Looking at the map, it appeared we were very close to being in Canadian waters. This we wanted to avoid, as the bureaucracy of our presence would keep all of us in red tape for months. It was Cliff who suggested he call for reinforcements, including a dog. We had Emma with the bad knee and One-Armed Jack, as well as the crotch man, all needing medical attention. We had a drug haul to make the DEA and Cliff heroes for a long time. Cliff was particularly convincing, saying a float plane would have us out of here in a few hours given the urgency. The idea of paddling back given how physically and emotionally exhausted I was feeling didn't seem all that rewarding. I appreciated that the exhaustion was in part a result of my conflicted roles of physician and gun-wielding avenger. The sidebar discussion, however, pointed out that if I was on the float plane, I would need to explain my presence here. John could easily get off as a guide, and while Mike might catch some bureaucratic heat, he would be okay. Mike offered to stay and help with the questions. He suggested that John and I canoe back and fish on the way. "You do have a fishing permit?" he asked. I had totally forgotten when getting the equipment. It would be my luck to get busted for that. We all laughed. John, Mike, and I collected Emma, and she and Mike returned to the group waiting for forest service officers, someone else from the DEA office, a tracking dog, and the float plane evacuation.

EPILOGUE

The float plane occupants quickly dispatched the wounded perpetrator in the woods after he tried to shoot the dog accompanying them. The wounded were evacuated and slowly recovered with some significant disabilities that did not evoke sympathy from the jury in their trial. Continued recovery is ongoing in a federal penitentiary. The bodies were taken to a morgue but were never claimed by any family members.

John and I made it out of the waters after a couple of leisurely days of canoeing and fishing. I managed to catch some nice walleye and northern. The simple, repetitive casting and reeling was amazingly therapeutic. Fortunately, we weren't stopped to check for a license, but as soon as we got to Ely, I purchased one. It seemed the right thing to do.

Tommy got through treatment and rejoined the practice after three months and continues with AA meetings and spot urine checks to prove sobriety as well as regular sessions with a therapist. He remains a great and gifted surgeon. He and Sue divorced but remain on friendly terms.

Capital Medical was raided by the DEA and police about the same time the float plane arrived to pick up Emma, One-Armed Jack, and Crotch Man. Jin was on the premises of Capital Medical and had in his possession some narcotics. This was an unfortunate mistake, as it was additive to his charges of narcotic distribution, smuggling, kidnapping, tax evasion, and more. His final sentence has yet to be determined.

Howard was arrested and charged with distribution. His cooperation led to additional charges against Jin. He was sentenced to thirty-six months in a federal penitentiary, this incarceration being served at a minimum-security facility near Pensacola, Florida, that is known for its relaxed rules; some have likened it to a club. It's still an incarceration. His son went on to play college baseball and unfortunately has not wished to see his father.

Kirk and Emma were reprimanded by the hospital administration, but—I believe based on my vouching for their character and professionalism, as well as there being a shortage of qualified perfusionists—they were allowed to keep their jobs. Their cooperation with the authorities also benefited their case at the hospital.

I returned to find the heparin debacle resolved with the closure, at least temporarily, of the Chinese manufacturing facility and the FDA enforcing more on-site management of foreign drug manufacturers. Our group received a thank-you from the FDA and an inquiry from a producer of *60 Minutes* about doing a story on the deadly heparin.

I recently received a call from Mike asking me to join him on a trip to Kenya next month. He mentioned a Chinese play on some natural resources and infrastructure in the area. He wanted my eyes. Who knows!

www.ingramcontent.com/pod-product-compliance
Lightning Source LLC
Chambersburg PA
CBHW020633220526
45464CB00001B/138